Do you or someone you love suffer from:

- Mild or severe depression?
- Sleepless nights?
- The pain of arthritis?
- Pain from fibromyalgia?
- Liver disease?
- Parkinson's disease?
- Alzheimer's disease?
- The side effects of prescription antidepressants?
- The frustration of not getting relief?

THE SAMe CURE
MAY BE THE RELIEF
YOU ARE LOOKING FOR!

THE
SAMe
CURE

DAN KLEIN

HarperTorch
An Imprint of HarperCollinsPublishers

THE SAMe CURE is not a substitute for sound medical advice. The ideas, procedures, and suggestions in this book are intended to supplement, not replace, the medical advice of a trained medical professional. All matters regarding your health require medical supervision. Consult your physician before adopting the suggestions in this book, as well as about any condition that may require diagnosis or medical attention. The author and publisher disclaim any liability arising directly or indirectly from the use of this book.

HARPERTORCH
An Imprint of HarperCollins*Publishers*
10 East 53rd Street
New York, New York 10022-5299

Copyright © 2000 by Dan Klein
ISBN: 0-380-81440-4

First HarperTorch paperback printing: August 2000

HarperCollins ®, HarperTorch™, and ◆ ™ are trademarks of Harper-Collins Publishers Inc.

Printed in the United States of America

Visit HarperTorch on the World Wide Web at www.harpercollins.com

OPM   10   9   8   7   6   5   4   3   2   1

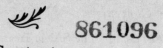

861096

Contents

FOREWORD by David W. Johnson, Ph.D.   *ix*

CHAPTER 1: "Cure du Jour" or Medical   *1*
            Breakthrough?

Part I: SAMe and Depression

CHAPTER 2: What Is Depression and   *13*
            Who Gets It?

CHAPTER 3: The Variety of Treatments   *33*
            for Depression

CHAPTER 4: Psychological Therapy   *39*
            for Depression

CHAPTER 5: Pharmacological Therapy for   *43*
            Depression: Prescription Drugs

CHAPTER 6: Pharmacological Therapy for   *51*
            Depression: "Natural"
            Antidepressants

CHAPTER 7: The SAMe Cure for Depression   *61*

Part II: SAMe and Arthritis

CHAPTER 8: Arthritis: What Is It and   *95*
            Who Gets It?

CHAPTER 9: The Most Common Treatments   *109*
            for Osteoarthritis

v

CHAPTER 10: The SAMe Treatment   *123*
             for Osteoarthritis

Part III: SAMe and Fibromyalgia

CHAPTER 11: Fibromyalgia: What Is It and   *143*
             Who Gets It?

CHAPTER 12: The Most Common Treatments   *151*
             for Fibromyalgia

CHAPTER 13: The SAMe Treatment   *159*
             for Fibromyalgia

Part IV: SAMe and Liver Diseases

CHAPTER 14: What Is Liver Disease and   *169*
             Who Gets It?

CHAPTER 15: The Most Common Treatments   *179*
             for Cirrhosis and Hepatitis

CHAPTER 16: The SAMe Treatment for   *183*
             Cirrhosis and Hepatitis

Part V: SAMe and Parkinson's Disease

CHAPTER 17: What Is Parkinson's Disease and   *195*
             Who Gets It?

CHAPTER 18: The Most Common Treatments   *199*
             for Parkinson's Disease

CHAPTER 19: The SAMe Treatment for   *205*
             Parkinson's Disease

Part VI: SAMe and Alzheimer's Disease

CHAPTER 20: What Is Alzheimer's Disease and   *211*
Who Gets It?

CHAPTER 21: Treatments for Alzheimer's Disease   *215*

CHAPTER 22: The SAMe Treatment for   *221*
Alzheimer's Disease

APPENDIX A   Buying SAMe   *225*

APPENDIX B   Further Information   *227*

INDEX   *229*

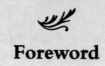

Foreword

There is no question among health-care professionals that Western medicine as we know it is in a state of transition. In the past 25 years, we have excelled in our ability to manage trauma, master extremely complex surgical techniques, develop much more sophisticated machinery to peer inside the body, and to treat disease more effectively once it exists. However, we have failed in the areas of actual disease prevention, as well as in managing the vast array of chronic incurable illnesses that are mostly age related and currently account for about 85% of the national health-care bill.

The predominate reason that we find ourselves in this medical quandary is our consistent failure to fund medical research on how to prevent or delay these chronic age-related diseases from occurring in the first place, at anywhere near the level that we fund research to treat disease after it exists. A report from the American Association of Naturopathic Physicians summed it up quite nicely, stating that "we wait for it [illness] to develop, and then we spend huge amounts of money on heroic measures, but ignore the underlying causes." This is analogous to waiting for your leaky roof to finally destroy your house, and then repairing the damage without fixing the leak.

This mentality still persists among many people in the health-care industry today for a number of reasons. At the top of the list is physician training. The fact remains that medical school curricula still consist almost entirely of learning anatomy and basic sciences in the first year, and then applying this to the diagnosis and treatment of disease in the clinical portion of the second year of didactic training. Students then spend two years rotating through clinical sites, where their primary job is to demonstrate this ability to diagnose disease and to prescribe the proper treatment. What little they may know about true disease prevention is brushed to the side, as they are well aware that it is only those students who can adequately demonstrate diagnostic and treatment skills for their preceptors who will pass clinical rotations.

There are other problems ingrained in the system as well. When medical students graduate and enter a residency program, they find themselves in a system that rewards rescue medicine, and intervention on existing disease. There is little reward, financial or otherwise, for physicians who take the time and trouble to try and prevent illness, or spend considerable time counseling their patients on adopting lifestyle changes that are healthy. This explains the huge popularity of the television series *ER* ("Emergency Room"), where physicians are often depicted knee deep in blood and guts, plugging the holes in gunshot victims and bringing them back from the brink of death, thus acquiring deity status. I can assure you that a proposed TV show titled *PR* ("Prevention Room"), which depicted physicians spending an hour with patients, counseling them about nutrition, supplements, exercise, or lifestyle changes they need to make to stay healthy would not make it to the pilot episode.

Other factors that work against physicians being advocates of disease prevention are time and money. Most new physicians come out of medical school with well over $100,000 of debt. Approximately 80% of doctors now practice in various health maintenance organizations (HMOs), for the simple reason that most insured patients now carry this type of health insurance. HMOs, once thought to be the only way to hold down the soaring costs in U.S. health care, have essentially made no one happy. One of the primary reasons that physicians dislike HMOs is that, to be profitable, the physician must see a large number of HMO patients each day. This dramatically cuts down the time the doctor can spend with her patients, and obviously increases the workload for the physicians. It is not uncommon for physicians in many practices to have to see patients every 15 minutes in order to be profitable, and this is simply not enough time for the physician to be able to adequately deal with most existing problems, much less discuss disease prevention.

Therefore, if physicians are largely untrained in preventive medicine after medical school, and if HMOs do not even give them enough time to sit down with healthy patients to discuss what they do know about maintaining health, who then is responsible for keeping you free of chronic disease for as long as possible? That's right: you. You the consumer have to take responsibility for your health maintenance by gathering information from reliable sources and working with your doctor with this information, to stay well as you age in years.

Daniel Klein has written an excellent book to help you in this endeavor. S-adenosylmethionine (SAMe) is a naturally occurring substance that has been studied extensively in humans, where it acts as a methyl donor in a large number of biochemical reactions. Donating a methyl group (i.e., "methylation") in biochemical reactions may not sound impressive to a layperson, but to scientists, the importance of this reaction in maintaining health cannot be overemphasized. Everything from activating or deactivating enzymes to converting the coded messages in our DNA to actual proteins involves methylation reactions, and therefore SAMe.

Clinical studies have long shown oral intake of SAMe to have antidepressant effects. Recent clinical studies have also shown it to be very effective in maintaining a healthy liver, and it is even effective in people who already have alcoholic liver cirrhosis. However, perhaps its greatest potential in preventing or delaying serious age-related disease lies in its ability to regulate plasma homocysteine metabolism. High levels of homocysteine, a sulfur-containing amino acid, have been highly correlated with the onset of cardiovascular and cerebrovascular disease. One very important way your body gets rid of homocysteine is to put a methyl group on it and form methionine, which is not harmful. SAMe is a major contributor to this process, and it does this by methylating a substance called tetrahydrofolate, which in turn methylates homocysteine to methionine. SAMe taken orally has been shown to increase levels of methylated tetrahydrofolate in humans, thus potentially decreasing their risk of cerebrovascular (stroke) and cardiovascular disease. This seems logical, when considered with the fact that patients with coronary artery disease have been shown to have significantly lower levels of SAMe than similar individuals without coronary artery disease.

SAMe may also have a role in cancer prevention. In certain types of cancer, reduced methylation of DNA may contribute to loss of the controls on genes that control normal cell division. In humans, low methylation of DNA has been observed in colorectal cancers and in their adenomatous polyp precursors. Low dietary folate and methionine and high intake of alcohol may reduce levels of SAMe, which as noted previously is required for DNA methylation. Therefore, oral supplementation of SAMe may be prophylactic in individuals at risk for these types of cancers.

Finally, as with many natural substances like SAMe, many will say, "If this stuff is so great, why isn't it a prescription drug that my doctor can provide?" The answer to this, of course, lies in the megaplex that is the pharmaceutical industry and its supposed regulator, the Federal Drug Administration (FDA). Briefly, the way the current system works is that pharmaceutical companies spend hundreds of millions of dollars testing a potential drug for many years, on animals on up to humans. They then submit the results of this testing to the FDA, where staff members are assigned to review the data. If it appears that the drug is relatively safe, and more effective than placebo, it gets approved (it doesn't matter if they don't have any idea exactly *how* the drug works). The pharmaceutical company gets a patent, which provides it exclusive rights to sell the drug for many years at a profit.

But this is truly an exclusionary process. First, only pharmaceutical companies have the facilities and command the type of cash, flow required to get a drug approved by the FDA. Additionally, naturally occurring substances (like SAMe) cannot be patented, so no one is going to invest hundreds of millions of dollars in getting FDA approval for a substance they cannot patent, even if preliminary evidence suggests it works. Therefore, most busy doctors will never have heard of substances like SAMe or have read the published clinical trials in which it was tested safely and effectively in humans. They are only required to know about the FDA-approved drugs on their formulary, and even what they know about these is generally the information provided by the parent drug company in the *Physician's Desk Reference*.

What this means, of course, is that a drug is neither safe nor effective until the FDA says it is safe and effective, and for the agency to say this, data costing hundreds of millions of dollars must be generated. This is not a horrible state of affairs, because we certainly need some type of regulation of products that are going to be introduced into use by physicians. But does this process really work? My opinion is that it does not work very well at all. Statistically, more than 50% of FDA-approved drugs are later found to have serious adverse affects not detected prior to approval, and some of these are fatal. In fact, an April 15, 1998, study in the *Journal of the American Medical Association* looked at hospital data and found that, in one year alone (1994),

FDA-approved drugs killed over 100,000 people and seriously injured more than 2 million others, and the authors concluded that "the incidence of serious and fatal adverse drug reactions in U.S. hospitals is extremely high." Given the fact that safety and efficacy data on drugs provided to the FDA for approval is produced by the drug companies themselves (and is therefore likely to be biased), and that a full-time staff of only around 50 individuals at FDA is responsible for monitoring the safety of over 5,000 brand-name, generic, and over-the-counter drugs after approval (when, as noted previously, many previously undetected serious side effects appear), are these numbers really surprising?

As you read this book, be aware that there are no miracle cures out there. But it is up to you the reader to understand how the medical model works, and as you can see, prevention of disease currently takes a backseat to the treatment of existing disease. Hopefully you also see that because a natural substance is not FDA approved does not necessarily mean that it is not safe and effective (although this may be the case), and that FDA-approved drugs are themselves not necessarily absolutely safe and effective. Understand that no pill will supplant the benefits of a healthy diet, regular exercise, and not smoking in staying free of chronic, incurable disease for as long as biologically possible. But there is mounting evidence that many natural substances can help in this process, and SAMe appears to be one of these.

David W. Johnson, Ph.D.
Associate Professor
Department of Pharmacology and
    Experimental Therapeutics
College of Osteopathic Medicine
University of New England

Adjunct Professor
Department of Physiology and
    Experimental Therapeutics
Boston University School of Medicine

ONE

"Cure du Jour" or Medical Breakthrough?

Medical "miracles" have been appearing on the market fast and furiously over the last 10 years. Melatonin, DHEA, St. John's wort, shark's fin cartilage, green algae—it is hard to keep count. And it's even harder to separate the medically tested preparations from the purely speculative ones.

The main reason that these new products are so hard for the consumer to judge is that federal laws governing their sale have recently changed, making it easier for new products to come on to the market (good), but also easier for these products to appear there without adequate experimental testing (not good.) Few, if any, of these new "miracle" products get onto drugstore and health-food store shelves without evidence that they are safe in moderate dosages. But whether they actually do any good—*whether they actually deliver what is promised*—frequently remains in question.

And now, along comes S-adenosylmethionine (SAMe), a naturally occurring molecule that is part of all living cells. It is being marketed as an expensive over-the-counter supplement that promises to cure—or at least significantly treat—a great number of the most prevalent and devastating diseases affecting Americans today. It is being touted as a virtual panacea, much the way the tonics and "snake oils" of the past were touted to unsuspecting and desperate consumers.

So the question is: Does SAMe actually deliver what it promises? And are there a substantial number of well-designed and executed, double-blind experimental studies that prove that it does?

The answer to both questions is a resounding yes!—at least for SAMe's most significant claims. And those include SAMe's efficacy in treating depression, osteoarthritis, cirrhosis of the liver, and fibromyalgia. (When it comes to Parkinson's disease and Alzheimer's disease, as we will see, the jury is still out, although preliminary data appears very promising indeed.)

How can one supplement have so many different beneficial effects?

SAMe's sheer variety of beneficial effects is certainly enough to make one suspicious—it sounds an awful lot like "snake oil," doesn't it? But the reason that SAMe affects so many different aspects of human biology and pathology lies in the fact that

SAMe operates on a fundamental biological process known as *methylation*—a process that occurs over a billion times per second throughout the body. Put simply, when a substance influences a process this basic—a process that is absolutely necessary for a number of critical life functions—it is bound to influence a great many vital aspects of the body.

Let's put that in another context. We all know that water is necessary for most basic life functions. And we know that if we are deprived of adequate amounts of water, every one of our body systems will slow down and finally stop functioning, resulting in sickness and eventually death. So there is a sense in which it could be said that adding water to a dehydrated person's diet "cures" a *huge* number of ailments, ranging from inadequate blood cell production to reduced brain function. That may sound a little simplistic, but the point is that when you are dealing with basic biological substances and basic biological processes, the effects are obviously going to be far-reaching.

There is something else we should consider when thinking about SAMe's multiple effects. Virtually *all* drugs and supplements have multiple effects, but these effects are broken down into the "primary effect" and the "side effect." The *primary effect* is the *intended* effect—the one for which you are taking the drug. A *side effect* is the unfortunate or unwelcome effect(s) that come along with the intended effect. For example, the primary or intended effect of taking an aspirin is reducing headache pain, while the frequent side effect is an upset stomach. Another example—one that becomes quite relevant when we compare Prozac with SAMe as a treatment for depression—is that one of the many possible side effects of Prozac is reduced libido and impotence in men. Certainly some patients have come to the conclusion that in the case of Prozac, the cure is worse than the disease—or, put another way, they would say that as far as they are concerned, *impotence* is the primary effect of Prozac.

Consider the drug minoxidil. When it was originally developed as a treatment for high blood pressure, researchers discovered that a frequent side effect of this drug was increased hair growth. Today, minoxidil is marketed as a hair restorer for bald people with the frequent and sometimes dangerous "side effect" of lowering the user's blood pressure!

The point is simply that the various effects of a given drug or supplement are either good or bad depending on what the desired effect of that drug is. For this reason, when referring to side effects, I identify those that reasonable people do not want as "unwelcome" side effects. So the bottom line is that, yes, SAMe has a great number of effects and, happily, most of these effects are quite welcome. In fact, one of the great advantages of SAMe treatment versus, say, Prozac, is that it has virtually no unwelcome side effects.

What is methylation?

We will be looking at what SAMe is and what the methylation process consists of from a variety of perspectives as we investigate SAMe's effects on different ailments. But let's lay down the basics here.

SAMe is a molecule that is a part of all living cells. Our bodies manufacture it from an amino acid called methionine, which is found in most proteins.

Methylation is a molecular transaction in which one molecule donates a four-atom part of itself to a nearby molecule. When this happens, both the donor molecule and the recipient molecule change shape, making huge differences in the way the human body conducts business. For example, methylation regulates DNA expression, insulates cells with protective membranes, and perhaps most significantly, regulates various hormones and neurotransmitters in our bodies. SAMe is by far the most active methyl donor in our bodies.

The chief way that the SAMe molecule changes after it has made its methyl donation to a neighboring molecule is that it becomes homocysteine, an extremely toxic substance that builds up in cells, causing untold damage unless our bodies recycle the homocysteine into the highest-ranking antioxidant in our bodies, glutathione. This latter process is called *remethylation*, a critical form of natural recycling. But unfortunately, this remethylation does not always happen or does not happen quickly enough to prevent homocysteine buildup and all the awful consequences of that molecular event.

The above may sound like gobbledygook to all but those of you who have recently taken biochemistry, but I believe it will all become much clearer as we investigate how SAMe and methylation influence individual body systems to cure or control individual ailments.

If SAMe is so effective, why don't all doctors routinely recommend it?

Unfortunately, the answer to this question is more of a political nature than of a scientific one. The basic reason doctors do not routinely recommend SAMe as a treatment—notably as a treatment for depression or osteoarthritis, where the scientific evidence for its efficacy is so strong—is simply because they do not know about it. Or they do not know enough about it to recommend it. Or perhaps what they do know about it has been given a negative "spin" by sources with a vested interest in keeping this drug from gaining popularity.

As any doctor will tell you, physicians are busy people. (That is why their waiting rooms are always full, right?) So most of the information that they receive about medical treatments and procedures after they have graduated from medical school is from two sources: medical journals and pharmaceutical company salespeople. There is no mystery why this latter source don't tell the doctors they visit about SAMe (or would be telling the doctors "bad" things about

SAMe). It is simply not in their economic self-interest; for one thing, expensive as SAMe is, prescription drugs that perform similar functions are more so. Add to this the fact that the drug companies give gifts like golf jaunts to the doctors they deal with. This could put a busy physician in a receptive frame of mind for listening to what they say (or don't say) about SAMe.

But what about the medical journals? Medical journals by and large have a conservative bias, tending to favor conventional treatments from conventional sources. And not to put too fine a point on it, most medical journals are dependent on advertising from pharmaceutical companies to pay their bills, so this may be reflected in the choices they make about which new medications to write about and which not to write about. Nonetheless, as we will see, many highly respected medical journals, both here and abroad, have published material about SAMe, most of it offering substantial evidence that SAMe is effective, particularly as a treatment for depression and osteoarthritis.

But why do some scientists insist that the scientific testing of SAMe is not up to standard?

First, not all of the testing *is* up to reasonable standards. The sample of subjects are often too small and the protocols of the testing procedures are often not rigid enough.

But that said, there remain a substantial number of finely made and executed tests of SAMe's efficacy in curing and treating various ailments. And, by and large, these are the tests I will be citing. Some scientists (particularly American scientists) will find even these studies lacking, but this may again be a result of a bias put out by the pharmaceutical companies.

In order to meet FDA standards for prescription drugs, these pharmaceutical megacorporations spend billions of dollars on exquisite tests, an expense that they say accounts for the high prices of their products. But in the opinion of more than one critic, these high-priced tests indulge in experimental overkill; they set test protocols and standards so high (and expensive) that no ordinary producer of over-the-counter preparations can match them. Does this mean that the test standards and test results that are less rigorous are always less than convincing to reasonable scientists? A growing number of scientists think not.

Finally, let me say a few words about how this book is set up. Each of its six parts is devoted to a disease that SAMe cures or treats (or, in the case of Parkinson's disease and Alzheimer's disease, *shows promise* of treating). We will start each part with a description of the particular disease and its causes; next we will look into both conventional and alternative treatments for this disease; and lastly we will look into how SAMe treats this disease and how this treatment compares with the others.

So if you are only interested in how SAMe deals

with one particular disease, turn to that section. However, you may want to check out sections in the other parts of the book that talk about how SAMe treats a particular disease in order to get a more complete picture of how this fundamental molecule influences the entire body.

PART I

SAMe and Depression

TWO

What Is Depression and Who Gets It?

What is depression?

In ordinary parlance, depression is a feeling of serious unhappiness over a sustained period of time—so much unhappiness that you cannot take pleasure in any part of your life. Nothing seems worth doing. And you don't have enough energy to do much of anything anyhow. One prominent psychiatrist defines depression as "the exact opposite of vitality."

This low feeling is often accompanied by feelings of personal worthlessness (extremely low self-esteem) and by feelings of excessive or inappropriate guilt, that is, guilt that no reasonable person would think you deserve to feel.

And along with these awful feelings, the following physical symptoms may occur: significant weight loss or gain (more than 5% either way in one month's time); insomnia (inability to sleep for a sufficient period of time or to sleep at all); general fatigue; headaches; and psychomotor agitation or retardation (restlessness or unusually slow movement).

Further, the following cognitive and behavioral symptoms may occur: diminished ability to concentrate and diminished ability to make decisions, even decisions of the simplest kind, like what to eat for breakfast.

In its most extreme form, depression is often accompanied by a preoccupation with death and with thoughts of suicide.

So you are saying there are degrees of depression?

Absolutely.

At one end is a single depressive episode—a few truly awful days when you don't enjoy anything, have low energy and zero motivation, think of yourself as a complete failure, and keep hitting yourself over the head for all the bad decisions you've made in your life and all the people you have let down. Yet a day or two later, life already looks a bit brighter, if not exactly filled with sunshine.

And at the other end is chronic severe depression—two years or more in which most of the awful feelings and many of the physical and behavioral symptoms mentioned above weigh you down without relief for longer than a month. It is at this end of the depressive spectrum that many people give up hope of ever feeling better again; in fact, a severely depressed person has virtually forgotten what it even feels like to be hopeful.

Psychiatrists deem the area in between these two extremes as moderate depression. Like the terms *middle class* and *average student*, the term *moderate depression* covers a huge area of territory and includes the great majority of people who believe they are suffering from some kind of depression.

Is there really a difference between being depressed and just being in a bad mood? Or is "depressed" just psychotalk for a really bad mood?

There is a difference, although it is more a difference of degree than of kind. The main difference lies in the intensity of the dark mood and in its duration and frequency. Further, most psychologists distinguish between an "accountable" bad mood and an "unaccountable" bad mood, calling only the latter a sign of depression.

First, let's consider *intensity*. We're wading into deeply subjective waters here, so drawing a line where "lousy mood" crosses over into "depressive episode" is fairly arbitrary and personal. One man's "funk" may be another man's "bout with severe depression." But that said, each of us pretty much knows when he's crossed his personal line from a bad mood to genuine depression: We simply can *feel* the difference. While that hardly qualifies as a scientific definition, I don't believe we need a tough-minded scientific definition for the *experience* of depression.

Duration of symptoms brings us back into a more objective area. Psychologists contend that a dark mood that never seems to end has crossed over into the realm of a psychological abnormality. If somebody said, "I've been in a bad mood for the last five years," we'd probably laugh. That's not a mood, we'd think, that's a way of life—a *depressive* way of life. Sure, it seems rather arbitrary that the American Psychiatric Association's definition of severe depression pins a precise number on duration (two or more years without relief for more than a month). But most of us can agree with the principle: If you are down that long and that relentlessly, you've got yourself a real problem—a problem that begs to be dealt with.

Frequency of symptoms falls into the same category as duration. If a person feels depressed a few days a week, week in and week out, she has crossed the line from a string of bad moods to a mood disorder. The commonsense principle is the same: If you are down that frequently for that long a time, you've got yourself a real problem—a problem that begs to be dealt with.

Finally, it makes good sense to distinguish between an accountable mood and an unaccountable mood disorder, drawing a line between the two by what, if anything, *causes* the emotion. If you have good reason for feeling blue—say, a death in the family—the resulting blue mood is considered accountable, appropriate, and thus acceptable. It is acceptable in the sense that it is just part of being human and grown up: When bad things happen we feel bad about them. That's the way it is and that's the way it should be. It is also acceptable in the sense that usually we would not seek psychological and/or pharmacological help to dissipate this accountable mood. (There are notable exceptions, of course. Many of us can benefit from grief counseling to adjust to extremely painful losses; but even then we do not expect to dissipate or short-circuit our feelings of grief, only to get through them the best we can.)

But if we experience bad moods for no apparent reason—that is, nothing unusually bad has happened to us recently and yet we still feel terribly low—it makes good sense to suspect that we are suffering from the mood disorder known as depression. In other words, You feel bad *in spite of* what is going on in your life rather than *because of* what is going on in your life.

But most people who are feeling blue always seem to give some *reason for it, don't they?*

True enough. When people feel down in the dumps they almost always *believe* that there is some outside cause of it.

"I feel lousy because I wasn't invited
to the Johnsons' for dinner";

or

"I feel lousy because I never save enough money";

or

"I feel lousy because I am overweight."

At the time we are experiencing this bad mood, these reasons (and thousands like them) seem like they must be the cause. But hold on: Couldn't we be confusing cause and effect? On other days, not being invited to the Johnsons' would not necessarily feel like a slight—in fact, it might very well feel like a relief. And on other days, our weight or financial status doesn't figure much in our consciousness at all because we have better—and happier—things on our mind. So why is this day different from those other days? Could it be because we are actually in an unaccountable bad mood—a bad mood without an immediate cause? Yet out of psychological habit, we *assign* a cause to our bad mood from the outer world. Heaven knows there is always *something* wrong out there if we need to find something wrong to account for our blues.

But who is to say what's a reasonable cause for being in a bad mood and what is not?

That's a tricky one, isn't it? The American Psychiatric Association (APA) only cites "death of a loved one" as a "normal" cause of a sustained accountable depressive mood. (They call it, rather unpoetically, "uncomplicated bereavement.") But why isn't loss of a job also included? Or infidelity of a spouse? Or losing your house in a poker game?

I am serious. Different folks value different things. Some of us may pin our entire identity and personal worth on our work, so if we lose our job we are so devastated we sink into an abysmal mood that lasts months, maybe even years. Now other people may think investing so much in our careers represents "bad values," values that cause us a lot of unnecessary pain. But who are they to say? Who, indeed, is to say what is a reasonable and accountable bad mood and what is a psychologically abnormal one?

I choose to sidestep this particular problem by suggesting a pragmatic approach, one that raises the only truly important question for people considering taking SAMe or any other medication/preparation in order to deal with unwelcome and distressing emotions: Would your overall life be significantly better if you didn't feel this way anymore?

If you answer yes to that question, you can proceed to the next step, namely, figuring out how you can best change the way you now feel, whatever term you choose to describe the way you now feel.

And if you answer no, well, good.

What is the cause of an unaccountable bad mood, then? In other words, what causes depression?

Traditional Freudian and neo-Freudian psychologists believe that the original cause of clinical depression in a person can be found in his childhood experiences. For example, many psychologists believe that a prime source of adult-onset depression is repressed anger in childhood; a child who is forever bottling up his anger will later in life experience depressive episodes or even chronic severe depression. Childhood traumas of various kinds—including physical and sexual abuse—are also thought to be an original cause of depression in both children and adults.

Depression is also a byproduct of anxiety disorders. Chronically anxious individuals often sink into depression because of their inability to cope with ordinary life situations.

But don't psychiatrists now know that there is a physical cause of depression—a chemical imbalance that causes it?

Not exactly. We now know that there is a chemical component to depression, but that is not the same thing as saying that the primary cause is chemical.

In the next chapter, we'll look in greater detail into

the chemistry of depression—what is going on in the brain and other parts of the nervous system that result in depressive feelings. But that particular chemical/neurological setup may itself be the result of psychological events. In other words, some childhood experiences or traumas may do something to the chemistry of the brain that predisposes it to depression at some later point in its development. If we think of it that way, the chemistry component is an intermediary step in the making of depression, but not the first cause.

In his seminal book *Listening to Prozac*, Dr. Peter Kramer posits the idea that stressful and unhappy psychological events in our early development cause "scars" in our neurological makeup, and then subsequent events in our lives "scrape" these scars, making them even more vulnerable to psychological injury—injury that is experienced as depression. It's the same idea: psychological events cause physical damage which, in turn, causes the psychological experience of depression.

Of course, like all nature vs. nurture arguments, this one gets more complicated when we introduce the role that genetics plays. Recent evidence strongly suggests that depression—even mild chronic depression—runs in families. In other words, there seems to be a genetic predisposition to depression in many cases. And if that is so, depression would seem to be a chemical matter. That is, it would seem that way until we realize that some members of the same family end up depressive while others do not. Is that because some got the "depressive gene" and others did not? Or is it because some "depressive genes" were triggered by traumatic psychological events and some were not? Genetic science is not at all clear on the answer to that one yet.

But is it really that critical to know what the first cause of our depression is—whether it is psychological or chemical (or both)? Or is the only important question what will cure it?

Once again, it makes good sense to think pragmatically. All we really need to know is how to cure our depression—wherever it came from.

It never ceases to amaze me how many people have a problem with this way of thinking. They say, "If depression has a psychological cause, then the only legitimate way to cure it is through psychological means—through talk therapy." The logic of this argument totally escapes me (although I do believe there can be benefits to talk therapy that antidepressants alone cannot provide—but more about that in Chapter 7).

Unfortunately, I *do* understand the politics of this argument. Psychologists without medical degrees cannot prescribe prescription antidepressants like Prozac. So it would hardly be in their interest to take the position that a pill could rid their patients of depression; at the very least, it could put a dent in their business (in fact, it already has). It will be interesting to see if psychologists will recommend some of the new non-prescription treatments for depression, like SAMe and St. John's wort, to their patients.

But isn't this so-called "pragmatic" approach opening the door to a feel-good mentality? Just about everybody wants to feel significantly better, but that doesn't mean they should take any feel-good medication/preparation that comes down the pike, does it?

Again, this is more of a values question than a psychological or medical one. But let me set the record straight on a few relevant facts.

First, taking SAMe (or Prozac or St. John's wort or any other clinically tested antidepressant) for unwelcome and distressing feelings will *not* set you on a road to excessive feel-good drug taking. You will *not* find yourself seeking out more powerful (and possibly dangerous) drugs or potions to make you feel even better. On the contrary, people who are considered chronically depressed by APA standards and who remain untreated are far more likely to end up taking a dangerous feel-good drug like cocaine than someone who has his depression under control by use of an antidepressant. People who are chronically depressed are often so desperate for relief from the pain of their depression that they will self-medicate with anything they can get their hands on to dull the pain, be it alcohol or a narcotic.

Second, most people who have a satisfying experience with antidepressants report that basically what makes them feel so much better is that they don't feel bad anymore: They no longer feel worthless, guilty, helpless, unmotivated, self-punishing, overtired, etc. And when they are released from all their negative feelings, their positive, life-affirming feelings get a chance to flourish.

This is a far cry from the detached feel-good high that narcotics and other controlled substances provide.

In a similar vein, people who have a satisfying experience with antidepressants often report that they feel "like themselves again." This sober-sounding experience sounds radically different from the dreamy, mystical, out-of-body feel-good experiences provided by narcotics and hallucinogens.

Most of us sense a legitimate difference between taking a pill so that we don't have to feel awful anymore and taking a pill just to get off and feel good. In the former instance, we are choosing more than just a new "mood," we are choosing a way to live our lives. In the latter, we are simply choosing to feel good for some time-limited period.

What do you mean when you say that by taking an antidepressant we are doing more than just changing our mood, we are choosing a way to live our lives?

I mean that chronic or recurrent depression is, sadly, a way of life—a joyless, unproductive, often isolating, and usually unloving way of life. And so when we choose to do something to end our depression, we are choosing a life that is the very opposite of that, a life that has a capacity for joyous experiences, productive activity, and loving relationships—all of which is far more than simply choosing to be in a better mood.

Freud said that the prime condition of mental health is the ability "to work and love." Well, it is virtually impossible for a chronically depressed person to pursue a successful career or to have satisfactory relationships with his mate or children.

How many people in the United States suffer from some form of depression?

According to American Psychiatric Association criteria, 50 million Americans suffer from some form of depression—that is approximately one out of every six people.

Just how does a person's depression affect the people around her?

Badly. Couples therapists will tell you that the single most destructive element in most relationships is one (or both) partner's depressive mood and behavior. A depressed person is often withdrawn and uncommunicative; a depressed person frequently has little or no sexual appetite; a depressed person is prone to drink excessively with concomitant aggressive drunken behavior; a depressed person is usually unable to empathize with anyone else's feelings. The list goes on, but the underlying problem remains the same: It is virtually impossible to enjoy your life for any length of time in the company of someone who has lost all capacity to enjoy her life.

And it gets worse. Because there is a sense in which depression is contagious. One psychiatrist I know told me that the best way he has for diagnosing depression in a new patient is by noting how he himself feels at the end of the hour: If he senses a heavy, claustrophobic, lifeless feeling lingering in himself, he is pretty sure the patient is depressed and brought his depression with him into the room.

It makes sense that if we are constantly in the company of a depressed person, we inevitably start to become depressed too. Some therapists have called this the "seductive power" of depression, but I think that misrepresents the fundamental dynamic. What is going on is a psychological variation of "If you can't lick 'em, join 'em"; if we cannot lift our partner out of her depression, cannot continually sustain our own good spirits around this person, and yet we want to stay connected to this person, we bring ourselves down to his depressed level. Now how is that for togetherness?

But looking at this phenomenon from the reverse direction, the news is very good indeed. If a depressed person gets out of his depression, his partner will start feeling a whole lot better too. In fact, some studies show that if one partner in a couple of two mildly depressed people is successfully medicated for his depression, the other partner will often experience relief from her depression too. Just like the disease, the cure is at least partially "contagious" too.

Are there different types of depression?

Yes, not only are there different degrees of depression—mild, moderate, and severe, as well as chronic and recurrent—there are also different types of depression. We should pay particular attention to three of these types: bipolar disorder (manic-depressive syndrome), seasonal pattern depression (seasonal affect disorder), and premenstrual syndrome (PMS) depression.

Bipolar disorder is marked by periods of manic feelings alternated with depressive periods. It is important to note that manic feelings are not merely good and happy feelings, they are grandiose, wildly out of touch with reality feelings. For example, in a manic phase of bipolar disorder, an individual may spend all his money (and then some) to fly his friends to the Caribbean for the weekend. It is the general case that the higher the manic phase, the deeper the depression that follows. (People with extremely severe bipolar disorder are more likely to contemplate suicide during their manic phase— when they know the big drop is on the way—than during the depressive phase itself.) The brain chemistry of bipolar disorder is somewhat different from the chemistry of the more common chronic depression and so responds better to different kinds and combinations of antidepressants. Psychiatrists do not recommend SAMe as the sole medication for bipolar disorder.

Seasonal affect disorder (or SAD) is a recently discovered and interesting variation on garden-variety low-grade depression: It is depression that comes in winter and improves in spring as the days lengthen. Most scientists agree that the prime cause of SAD is the scarcity of sunlight in winter—that, in fact, our nervous system needs sunshine to promote melatonin production which, in turn, promotes other chemical responses that keep depression at bay. (These scientists point to the high incidence of depression and suicide in extremely northern countries like Sweden, where the sun shines for as little as two hours a day in midwinter.) Basically, SAD's brain chemistry is similar to that of most normal-range depressions. Some people prefer to treat it with melatonin supplements and/or regular exposure to artificial broad-spectrum light, which mimics sunshine, but it responds at least equally as well to antidepressants like Prozac and SAMe.

Premenstrual syndrome depression has been well known to women for a very long time, but only recently has it been recognized by the psychological community at large. (Sadly, women's mental health problems have generally been given short shrift by the male-dominated psychiatric community.) Because this particular type of depression is time-limited to no more than one week out of four, most women who suffer from it elect not to medicate with antidepressants. (Antidepressants, including SAMe, only work if they are taken continuously over a period of time; they cannot help if only taken on "bad" days or weeks.) Nonetheless, women who suffer severely from PMS depression have found relief by taking antidepressants, including SAMe, all of the time.

Are some people more likely to suffer from depression than others?

Yes. Statistically, women are more likely to suffer from depression than men, and postmenopausal women and new mothers (postpartum depression) are at particular risk. People over 65 of either sex are more likely to suffer from depression than younger people, and the risk of depression increases as a person gets older than 65. People with chronic debilitating illnesses are highly prone to depression, both as a result of the "accountable" sadness that comes from being incapacitated and of the weakened ability of the relevant parts of the immune system to fight off depression. Finally, people with a history of depression in their families are more likely to suffer from depression than those without such a history.

But that still leaves literally millions of people who do not fit into any of the above categories, yet who suffer, in one degree or another, from depression. And they are rich and poor, young and middle-aged, educated and uneducated, married, single, gay . . . you name it. As one of my colleagues says, "Depression is an equal-opportunity disease."

Can you be depressed without realizing it?

Oh, yes. The Danish philosopher Søren Kierkegaard said that the very essence of despair is that it is unaware of itself. In fact, the more seriously depressed you are, the less likely you are to realize that you suffer from depression. One reason for this is that chronic, long-term depression becomes the only reality you know. Deep depression starts to feel like regular life—as the late writer Richard Fariña titled his book, *Been Down So Long It Seems Like Up to Me*. A related reason for a seriously depressed person's lack of consciousness of his condition is that depression kills his capacity for hope: He literally cannot imagine feeling differently in the future. So he doesn't think he is depressed, he just thinks that this is the way life is.

Can you tell if someone else is depressed, even if he doesn't think that he is?

Yes. You can often tell by a person's tone of voice (flat, unenthusiastic), by his body language (stooped, lethargic movements), by his facial language (downcast eyes, dull, lifeless expression), and by his general attitude (pessimistic, relentlessly negative). Like my psychiatrist friend mentioned above, you may also be able to tell by how the person makes you feel after spending time with him: If you feel a transient depression, it may be the result of "catching" his.

You may also be able to tell by the person's emotional behavior (crying spells, extreme irritability), by changes in her eating habits (either compulsive eating or complete loss of appetite), by changes in the way she relates to other people (withdrawn, nonsexual), and by changes in the way she approaches work (neglects responsibilities). Finally, there may be purely physical clues (trembling extremities, slowed reflexes).

But I would strongly advise against telling anyone that you think she is depressed, even if the evidence is overwhelming. Your motives for telling her may be pure and altruistic, but you are not likely to help her by your pronouncement; on the contrary, you are more likely to make her withdraw even further.

Then what can you do to help if you are pretty sure that someone is depressed and you are also pretty sure that he doesn't realize it?

I think the best thing to do is leave gentle hints around his environment—books and articles about depression and its cures (including the SAMe cure) that discuss it sympathetically and clearly.

THREE

The Variety of Treatments for Depression

What are the major treatments for depression?

At the beginning of the twenty-first century, there are two major areas of treatment: psychological (mostly various types of "talk" therapy) and pharmacological (antidepressant medications or supplements). The great majority of Americans and Europeans who seek help in relieving their depression end up using one or both of these types of treatment.

For people suffering from extremely severe chronic depression, two other types of treatment are currently in use: surgical intervention (frontal lobotomy—removal of the frontal lobe of the brain) and electroconvulsive therapy (ECT, known as "shock therapy"—electrically induced mini-seizures that appear to "reset" the brain). Both of these treatments have severe and often permanent side effects; for that reason they are treatments of last resort for severe and intractable depression.

I would be remiss if I did not mention some other, less popular types of treatment for mild and moderate depression that have proven effective for at least some segments of the population.

Many depressed people have found relief via spiritual counseling from pastoral counselors. Like much of psychological "talk" therapy, spiritual counseling allows the depressed person to talk about his feelings in a nonjudgmental atmosphere and to put his feelings in a broader context, in this case a spiritual context. In fact, organized religion in the Western world has a long history of helping adherents rid themselves of uncontrollable distressing feelings, feelings that may not have been called depression at the time, but had remarkably similar symptoms. One way that organized religion once helped a person rid himself of his unwanted feelings was by exorcism—the source of the feelings were traced to an extraneous evil being that had taken possession of the ailing person's soul; the exorcism forced this evil being out. Say what you will, but for true believers it often worked as well as psychotherapy works today. Another way that organized religion helped (and still helps) some people rid themselves of their unwanted feelings was via prayer—prayer for relief and redemption. Again, for true believers, it had (and has) a pretty good record.

Today, some philosophers have hung out a shingle

to offer people help in dealing with personal problems, including depression. "Plato Instead of Prozac," one practitioner advertises. Instead of offering a spiritual perspective or context to put one's problems in, they offer a rational/philosophical perspective. It is too early yet to tell how effective this kind of treatment is; I admit to serious doubts about its effectiveness with anything but the mildest degrees of depression.

Eastern religious practices by Westerners have had some encouraging results for sufferers of mild depression. In particular, yoga and meditation, when practiced regularly, have a good record for bringing relief from some of depression's most common symptoms, including insomnia, fatigue, and psychomotor disorders. Studies have shown that yoga and/or meditation can significantly alter such measurable phenomena as brain waves and brain chemistry (which gives us one more spin to the puzzle of which came first, the psychological event or the brain chemistry), so even nonspiritual skeptics can appreciate the healing powers of these practices. In his book, *The Relaxation Response*, Harvard psychologist Herbert Benson shows that regular meditation engenders tranquilizing alpha brain waves, reducing overall stress to the nervous system. Thus far, yoga and meditation have proven more effective in dealing with anxiety disorders than with moderate or severe depression.

Isn't exercise good therapy for depression too?

It certainly can help, yes. A regular regime of plain old-fashioned physical exercise (jogging, swimming, biking, etc.) is proving to be a terrific hedge against low-grade depression. At first, psychologists believed exercise reduced symptoms of depression for merely psychological reasons—exercise provides balance in a stressed and depressed person's life and takes his mind off of his mind, so to speak. But recent studies have shown that there is a chemical component to this phenomenon too: Sustained exercise substantially increases production of brain chemicals called endorphins, and endorphins have a pain-relieving and a stress-releasing effect, both of which reduce the "pain" of mild depression.

How about diet and lifestyle—can't they help combat depression?

Without a doubt. One way of combating depression is by staying in good general health—a healthy immune system goes a long way in keeping depression at bay. This is probably why substantial intake of vitamin C has been demonstrated to help control mild depression. Also, inasmuch as chronic illness is closely associated with depression for both psychological and physical reasons, a healthy diet is obviously a good hedge against that type of depression.

Lifestyle is one of those words that seems to take on a different meaning depending on what magazine you are reading. In *Cigar Aficionado*, it means the good life of expensive clothes, cars, vacation spots, and, of course, cigars; in the *Vegetarian Times*, it clearly means something quite different. When it comes to describing a lifestyle that helps avoid and/or combat depression, our definition lies somewhere between the two. Obviously, a physically healthy lifestyle with a good diet, exercise, and *no* cigars is part of a basic "antidepressant" lifestyle. But some evidence also indicates that an aesthetically rich lifestyle with good music, tasty foods, and beautiful things to look at has antidepressant qualities too. No surprise here: it is difficult to keep up your capacity for pleasure if there is nothing pleasant available in your environment. Still, once a person has crossed the line into moderate or chronic depression, it doesn't seem to matter what pleasant and beautiful things are out there; the capacity to enjoy them is gone.

Are you suggesting that for most cases of depression, psychological and pharmacological therapies are more effective than the less popular therapies?

Yes, that definitely seems to be true for most people.

FOUR

Psychological Therapy
for Depression

What exactly is psychological therapy for depression and how does it work?

The basic form of psychological therapy is what is called "talk" therapy—therapy in which the patient talks to the therapist about his feelings, his personal history, and, often, his dreams; and the therapist offers the patient insights into why he feels the way he does. The therapist may also offer the patient advice on alternative ways to perceive people and events, and alternative ways to act in the world—ways that may help the patient detach from his depression and/or avoid events that trigger his depression. (A notable exception to this kind of talk therapy is classical Freudian psychoanalysis, in which the therapist says little or nothing to the patient, allowing him to dig into his feelings without judgment or interruption.)

There are various theories of how talk therapy

relieves depression, some of them fairly straightforward, some more subtle and complex. At the straightforward end is the notion that by talking about your bad feelings in a nonjudgmental, totally supportive environment, you "ventilate" them—that is, you expel them from your system. (In theory, at least, this is not so different from "exorcism.") Also at the straightforward end is the idea that, with the therapist's help, the patient is able to see connections between events in her life (particularly in her childhood) and her depressed feelings; and by seeing these connections, she is able to "detach" from them. For example, over the course of talk therapy a patient may realize that a prime source of her depression is that her mother always criticized and undervalued her, making her feel like a failure; but once she fully realizes that nothing she could have done (or could do now) would satisfy her mother, she is able to "detach" from this dynamic, to leave it and her depression behind her and to get on with her life.

At the more abstract end of the spectrum is the theory that by emotionally reliving traumatic childhood events as an adult (as compared to merely remembering them), the patient can neutralize the events, releasing him from the original cause of the depression. A key part of this theory is what Freud called "transference"; the patient transfers his feelings about his parent, to the therapist, then works through his childhood feelings about this parent by projecting them onto the therapist.

In recent years, psychoanalytic and psychothera-peutic theory have come under increasing attack for their unscientific basis. For example, it is virtually impossible to prove scientifically exactly what "reliv-ing a traumatic childhood event" is and, whatever it is, how it neutralizes depression. Mental and emo-tional events are not the sort of thing we can look at under a microscope or weigh on a scale. But pragma-tists like myself don't really care whether psychoana-lytic theory is scientifically provable or not. All we want to know is, does it work? Can talk therapy cure depression?

And the answer to that is a very qualified yes. In studies of groups of people with similar depressive symptoms and diagnoses, those who underwent a year or more of talk therapy were more likely to report some relief of their symptoms than those who had not undergone talk therapy. But the cure rate is nowhere near as impressive as the cure rate with many antidepressant medications.

Further, the duration of effective talk therapy often exceeds three years. Predictably, the more intense and chronic the depression, the lower is talk therapy's rate of success.

Aren't there other types of psychological therapy that do not involve just talk or do not involve talk at all?

Yes, there are a whole range of nonverbal psycho-logical therapies that are used in an effort to cure depression, ranging from Wilhelm Reich's Orgone Box (a wooden affair that the patient sits in while "bad energy" seeps out of him) to primal scream therapy (reliving the "original trauma" of birth). In between are various massage and body work therapies (Rolfing, the Alexander method, bioenergetics). All claim some success in curing depression; few have been studied thoroughly for success rates. Most mainstream mental health professionals believe that these types of therapy only work for a relatively small percentage of people who suffer from depression.

FIVE

Pharmacological Therapy for Depression: Prescription Drugs

What is pharmacological therapy for depression and how does it work?

Fundamentally, pharmacological therapy for depression is ingesting on a regular basis a chemical substance that alters the chemistry of the brain and which, in turn, relieves the symptoms of depression. When pharmacological therapy is successful, the pain of depression goes away, along with it the feelings of worthlessness and inappropriate guilt. Some or all depressive symptoms are lessened or go away completely: fatigue, insomnia, psychomotor problems, headaches, and the inability to concentrate and make decisions.

In itself, pharmacological therapy does *not* provide its user with any insights into her personality or how she came to suffer from depression in the first place. However, by significantly reducing the symptoms of depression, pharmacological therapy can signifi-

cantly alter the outlook, relationships, productivity—
even the personality—of its user.

Although different antidepressant chemicals work
in different ways, all of them work on the brain's neurotransmitters, in particular the neurotransmitters
norepinephrine, serotonin, and dopamine.

Hold on, what are neurotransmitters?

The brain is made up of billions of cells called *neurons*, and these neurons make contact with one
another via chemical messengers called *neurotransmitters*. Because the fundamental work of the brain—
thinking, remembering, feeling—is conducted by
connecting one neuron to another, neurotransmitters
are the basic stuff of brain activity.

After a neurotransmitter has done its duty as a
messenger, it is either recycled (used again by a neuron as a chemical messenger) or eliminated from the
body as a waste product. The efficiency with which
the brain recycles neurotransmitters accounts for
both the balance and the sum total of transmitters
hanging out in the brain at any given time. If the recycling is inefficient, the brain ends up with a net loss
of neurotransmitters. Both the relative balance of different neurotransmitters and the total population of
neurotransmitters have a pronounced effect on mood.
The wrong balance or too little of certain neurotransmitters contribute to all the major symptoms of
depression.

Are there different types of chemical products used to treat depression?

Yes. Basically, there are two types: prescription antidepressants and "natural" antidepressants. The former are chemical preparations that do *not* occur naturally in either the human body or in plants, and that require a doctor's prescription to acquire. The latter are substances that *do* occur naturally in either the human body or in plants, and that can be acquired over the counter. Ultimately, these definitions are more legal descriptions (following FDA guidelines for what can be sold over the counter and what cannot) than scientific ones. For example, although SAMe occurs naturally in the human body, the preparations of it that are sold over the counter in stores are manufactured synthetically.

What are the principal prescription antidepressants?

There are three main kinds: tricyclics, monomine oxidase (MAO) inhibitors, and selective serotonin reuptake inhibitors (SSRIs). Let's consider them one at a time.

TRICYCLICS

Tricyclics (so-called because of their three-ring chemical structure) are the oldest prescription antidepressants we have, so old that the patents on many of them have expired; hence, they are now available in generic (relatively inexpensive) form. The most commonly prescribed tricyclics are desipramine, imipramine, amitriptyline, doxepin, and nortriptyline. Although it has never been demonstrated exactly how they work, tricyclics raise the levels of two neurotransmitters in the brain, norepinephrine and serotonin. In depressed people, these two neurotransmitters are in short supply; however, if levels of norepinephrine and serotonin are boosted, many of the symptoms of depression vanish.

Tricyclics can be highly effective antidepressants, especially for depressives who have accompanying sleep disorders. Generally speaking, it takes about a month of regular doses of a tricyclic before there is a significant remission of depression.

But for a high number of people, tricyclics exact a terrible price for the good they do. The common, undesirable side effects of this prescription drug include blurred vision, constipation, urinary retention (inability to completely empty bladder), dry mouth, and unusual weight loss or gain (which is itself a symptom of depression!). Just slightly less common are general dizziness and a "drugged out" feeling. Also common are various sex-related hormone disorders: in men, swelling of the testes, development of breasts, and lowered sexual drive; in women, change in the shape of breasts and lowered sexual drive. It gets worse—possible seizures, irregular heart rhythms—but already there are enough side effects to make most of us seriously wonder if the cure may not be worse than the disease.

MAO INHIBITORS

Monoamine oxidase (MAO) inhibitors go a different route for a similar effect on neurotransmitters. An enzyme produced in the brain and the liver, MAO metabolizes (breaks down to release energy for body functions) norepinephrine, serotonin, and dopamine. So, when the MAO enzyme is inhibited, more of these three neurotransmitters survive, keeping the population of them in the brain up. The end result again is relief of depression. The most commonly prescribed MAO inhibitors are isocarboxazid, phenelzine, and tranylcypromine.

A small number of depressives do not respond to any antidepressant other than MAO inhibitors. These days such people are virtually the *only* ones taking MAO inhibitors because once again the price in unwelcome side effects is formidable. When combined with tyramine-rich foods, MAO inhibitors can raise norepinephrine levels to a point where the patient's blood pressure goes off the scale, putting him at serious risk for sudden death from hypertension. This would not be so bad if the list of tyramine-rich foods was not so extensive—cheese, yeast, wine, beer, pickled foods, chicken livers, coffee, soy and other bean products, just for starters. Yes, one can do without all of these foods, but the possible danger of one of them being an undetectable part of some recipe makes eating anywhere but home an extremely risky business.

SSRIs

Finally, there are the selective serotonin reuptake inhibitors (SSRIs), the newest generation of prescription antidepressants and by far the most popular today. Yes, we're talking about the wonder drug that has taken America by storm, Prozac (fluoxetine)! We are also talking about Prozac's successors, Zoloft (sertraline), Paxil (paroxetine), Luvox (fluvoxamine), Effexor (venlafaxine), and Celexa (citalopram).

Basically, SSRIs work like the tricyclics—they boost the brain population of the neurotransmitter serotonin by improving the efficiency with which it is recycled by brain neurons. And once more that serotonin boost means a decrease in the symptoms of depression. (There can, however, be too much of a good thing: An overabundance of serotonin can lead to manic symptoms and behavior.) In general, SSRIs take about three or four weeks of steady dosage to reach maximum effect.

For some people, Prozac also has beneficial psychological "side effects": it helps control some eating disorders and obsessive-compulsive disorder. But once again, the *unwelcome* side effects are daunting, to say the least. Nausea, headaches, and insomnia are fairly common for people taking this drug. A little further down the scale are diarrhea, muscle weakness, loss of appetite, tremors, dizziness, night sweats, and dry mouth. Perhaps most distressing is the all-too-common side effect of decreased sexual appetite and, in a striking number of cases in both men and women, the inability to reach orgasm. Not an awful lot of pleasure available here, even if your capacity for pleasure has been restored.

SIX

Pharmacological Therapy for Depression: "Natural" Antidepressants

What are the major "natural" antidepressants and how do they work?

First, let me clarify that by "natural" antidepressant, I simply mean those antidepressant preparations that you can get over the counter in your health food, nutrition, and drug stores—that is, you can purchase them *without* a prescription. Prescription drugs are *usually* synthetic substances that do *not* occur naturally in the human body or in plant form, but this is not always the case (e.g., insulin occurs naturally in the human body, but insulin supplements require a prescription). So I will leave the distinctions between "natural" and "unnatural" to the Food and Drug Administration (FDA) and simply get on with a description of the major nonprescription antidepressants.

The principal over-the-counter preparations that have demonstrated some antidepressant capabilities include St. John's wort, melatonin, kava-kava, valerian root, L-tryptophan and 5-HTP, Acetyl-L-Carnitine, and SAMe.

What is St. John's wort and how does it work as an antidepressant?

St. John's wort (*Hypericum perforatum*) is an herb that has been used as a remedy for anxiety and sleep disorders since the pre-Christian era. Currently, it is the antidepressant of choice by the majority of German doctors, and is growing quickly in popularity in the rest of Europe and in the United States. Like the major prescription antidepressants, St. John's wort treats depression by boosting the brain population of the neurotransmitters serotonin, dopamine, and nor-epinephrine, although how it achieves this effect is still unknown. It may also lower levels of the stress hormone cortisone.

Because of its popularity in Germany, St. John's wort has been the subject of many thorough controlled studies (as many, to date, as have been performed on Prozac), and all of them indicate a high cure rate for mild depression. In general, it takes a steady dosage of St. John's wort for four to six weeks to reach maximum effectiveness. Just what comprises an appropriate dose is hard to determine. Most people start with a dose 300 milligrams three times a day and work up or down from there after taking it the initial six weeks. (People eager to find relief from depression may find this is an awfully long period to wait in order just to determine whether or not the dosage is right.) Recent evidence indicates that a dosage of higher than 300 milligrams is needed by most people to match the effects of a standard dose of Prozac.

St. John's wort is far less expensive than any of the prescription drugs; further, it does not require expensive visits to psychiatrists or other M.D.s in order to acquire a prescription. So why isn't St. John's wort the antidepressant of choice of everyone in this country?

Two reasons: First, St. John's wort has a number of unwelcome side effects too—side effects that, for example, SAMe does not have. And second, like other over-the-counter preparations—including SAMe—St. John's wort is not regulated or monitored by the FDA. And that means that the purity and concentration of any particular preparation you buy at any particular time is not necessarily consistent. Actually, this is an argument against using any over-the-counter preparation!

Let's look at St. John's wort's most common side effects. They include sexual dysfunctions, nausea, diarrhea, nervousness, sleepiness, and tremors. Oops, sounds a lot like Prozac, doesn't it?

What is melatonin and how does it work as an antidepressant?

Melatonin is a hormone that is produced naturally in the pineal gland of humans and whose chief function is to set and maintain our internal biological clock and sleep cycle. As melatonin is a natural end product of metabolizing the neurotransmitter serotonin, a deficiency of melatonin is frequently associated with depression—particularly age-related depression and seasonal affect disorder (SAD).

Both of these cases are relatively easy to account for. First, our natural production of melatonin decreases with age (by the time we are 60, we only have half as much of it circulating in our systems as we did at 25), causing a deficiency in our later years that may induce depression. Second, although direct sunlight blocks the production and release of melatonin into the bloodstream, exposure to sunlight is necessary to "prime" the pineal gland for production of melatonin at night. So, in the months when the sun does not shine much (and we do not go outside often), we are likely to experience a melatonin deficiency and the depression associated with this deficiency. Thus, it comes as no surprise that at least for these two types of depression, melatonin supplements seem to offer an effective and inexpensive cure. Also, inasmuch as melatonin supplements produce deep and restful sleep, and there is nothing like a good night's sleep to tame a mild depression, common sense tells us that it can help in this regard. (Some people combine diurnal doses of St. John's wort or other antidepressants with doses of melatonin at night.)

Appropriate dosage of melatonin is highly individual. It is generally suggested that you start with a .5 milligram dose a half hour before bedtime and increase that dosage by .5-milligram increments until you find the right amount to put you into a deep and restful sleep for eight hours without a drowsy "hangover." Such drowsiness, by the way, is the only significant unwanted side effect I know of. But it is one reason why one should be careful driving and operating heavy machinery until you know your tolerance for this supplement.

So, in general we can say that melatonin appears to be an inexpensive and relatively side effect–free supplement that helps control certain types of mild depression, but that is about all we can say for sure at this point. Although many controlled studies have been made on melatonin's efficacy as a treatment for sleep disorders and jet lag (all with convincing results), there have not been a sufficient number of studies of melatonin's efficacy as a treatment for depression to make an unqualified recommendation of its use as an antidepressant.

What is kava-kava and how does it work as an antidepressant?

Kava-kava or kava root (*Piper methysticum*) is an herb that grows in the South Sea Islands and has been used by the native populations there for centuries as a medicine, religious libation, and what we would call a recreational drug. (In these native cultures, there is often little or no distinction between medication and recreation—perhaps not such a bad idea for our own culture that is awash with stress-induced ailments.) As a medication, kava-kava is used by islanders to promote sleep, ease pain, cure infections, calm the stomach, cure headaches—the list is long and impressive.

In our own culture, kava-kava is used chiefly to reduce anxiety and treat insomnia. And inasmuch as anxiety disorders often translate into depressive disorders (see Chapter 2), kava-kava is also used to treat anxiety-related depression. Almost all the studies on kava-kava's effectiveness in treating psychological disorders have been done in Europe, most of them using "self-reporting" subjects who grade themselves on anxiety and mood scales before taking kava-kava and then after taking either it or a placebo. The results clearly indicate a reduction of anxiety symptoms and of depression that is associated with anxiety. They also indicated no significant side-effects other than drowsiness. Two German scientists who studied the herb, Drs. Hans-Peter Volz and M. Kieser, went so far as to declare that based on the results of their study, they believed that kava-kava was "a treatment alternative to tricyclic antidepressants and benzodiazepines in anxiety disorders, with proven long term efficacy and none of the tolerance problems associated with tricyclics and benzodiazepines."

What is valerian root and how does it work as an antidepressant?

Like kava-kava, Valerian Root (*Valeriana officinalis*) is a time-honored herbal folk remedy that is used primarily to treat insomnia and reduce anxiety. For most homeopathic physicians in the United States, it is prescribed to address the same symptoms for which conventional doctors prescribe Valium. And again, inasmuch as anxiety disorders often translate into depressive disorders, valerian root is also used to treat anxiety-related depression. At the present time, there have not been a sufficient number of studies of valerian root's efficacy as a treatment for anxiety-related depression to make an unqualified recommendation of its use as an antidepressant.

What are L-tryptophan and 5-HTP and how do they work as antidepressants?

L-tryptophan is an essential amino acid found in some foods (turkey, beef, soy) that is a *precursor* of the neurotransmitter serotonin—that is, L-tryptophan is naturally transformed in the human body into serotonin. For that reason, loading up on L-tryptophan via either food or supplements results in increased serotonin production, raising the overall brain population of that antidepressant-acting neurotransmitter. This amino acid is extremely effective as a soporific (sleep aid) and also has a good record alleviating mild anxiety and mild depression. Unfortunately, L-tryptophan is currently off the market, allegedly because of a contaminated batch of supplements that caused several people to become seriously ill. (The accepted wisdom in many circles is that this relatively inexpensive and unpatentable amino acid was removed from the market to accommodate major pharmaceutical companies who were marketing more expensive competing products such as the soporific Halcion.)

The good news, however, is that a modified form of L-tryptophan called 5-HTP (5-hydroxytrytophan) has recently arrived on the market. (5-HTP is manufactured from seeds of the plant *Griffonia simplicifolia*, whereas L-tryptophan is produced by a biofermentation process.) 5-HTP is an even closer precursor of serotonin and therefore loading up on 5-HTP significantly boosts the serotonin population in the brain. According to the first few studies, 5-HTP appears to compare favorably with both tricyclics and SSRIs in treating mild and moderate depression.

What is more, 5-HTP appears to have only two significant common side effects. The first is that, like L-tryptophan, it causes drowsiness, thus making it a fine sleeping pill, but dangerous to take before driving or using other heavy machinery. The second is that it curtails craving of carbohydrates with the end result of causing weight loss, not an unwelcome side effect for many users.

But once again, because over-the-counter preparations do not require e×ːⱨ̣. ʳe (and expensive) testing as long as they do not make specific health claims,

5-HTP has not been sufficiently tested as a treatment for depression to make an unqualified recommendation of its use as an antidepressant.

Nonetheless, this amino acid is a supplement that many find to be very promising as an inexpensive and effective "natural" antidepressant with negligible side effects. I believe 5-HTP is well worth keeping an eye on as more studies of it trickle in.

What is Acetyl-L-Carnitine and how does it work as an antidepressant?

Acetyl-L-Carnitine (ALC) is a naturally occurring molecule involved in the transport of fats into the mitochondria (the energy-producing parts of cells) that is used medically primarily as a "smart drug" (nootropic)—that is, it is used to enhance cognitive functions like memory, problem solving, and eye-hand coordination. ALC has proven particularly helpful in stemming age-related memory loss, including both senility and Alzheimer's disease. Although it has not been proven conclusively, it is thought that ALC enhances and protects cognitive functions by intensifying the activity of the enzyme acetylcholine and/or by increasing neurol metabolism. There is also evidence that ALC supplements boost production of the neurotransmitter dopamine.

In several Italian studies, ALC has also been found to significantly reduce symptoms of depression in older people (between ages 60 and 80). Most scientists believe this is because of the dopamine boost. But several psychologists have weighed in with a rather commonsense explanation: because the fundamental cause of age-related depression is the decline of cognitive abilities (and the person's *consciousness* of this loss), improving these cognitive abilities has a logical antidepressive effect! Further, ALC was found to improve the quality of sleep in this population, a phenomenon that also naturally reduces depression.

Altogether, no significant side effects were found in taking the normally effective dose of ALC (3,000 mg). Therefore, for age-related depression—particularly depression in older people with cognitive deficits—Acytel-L-Carnitine is strongly recommended as a "natural" antidepressant.

Many people believe that other over-the-counter nootropics such as ginkgo biloba and deprenyl are equally successful as ALC in treating age-related depression, but neither one has been sufficiently tested as a treatment for age-related depression to make an unqualified recommendation of its use as an antidepressant.

What is SAMe and how does it work as an antidepressant?

This question deserves a chapter of its own—the next one.

SEVEN

The SAMe Cure for Depression

What is SAMe and how does it work as a treatment for depression?

S-adenosylmethionine (SAMe) is a molecule that is produced in *all* living cells, including human cells. We produce it from a substance called adenosine triphosphate (ATP) and an amino acid called methionine, which is found in protein-rich foods and is considered to have properties that affect both mood and cognitive functions. When our cells produce a sufficient number of SAMe molecules, an essential substance called a methyl group is released, which in turn fuels dozens of biochemical reactions in our bodies. This process, known as methylation, happens over a billion times per second throughout our bodies, and is necessary for a variety of fundamentally important life functions ranging from fetal development to brain operation.

Methylation is also critical in the regulation of certain hormones, including the stress hormone adrenaline and certain neurotransmitters, including melatonin, serotonin, and dopamine. Here, as with the prescription tricyclic and SSRI antidepressants, is the primary way SAMe affects mood/depression—by boosting the ongoing brain population of these neurotransmitters.

There are two salient facts that demonstrate the relationship between SAMe and depression: SAMe levels decrease significantly in people suffering from depression. Of course, this in itself does not prove that raising SAMe levels will decrease symptoms of depression, but numerous studies now demonstrate just that: Raise SAMe levels and symptoms of depression decrease or go away altogether.

And when it comes to raising those SAMe levels circulating in our cerebrospinal fluid, there is clear-cut evidence that SAMe supplements—administered either orally or intravenously—are capable of crossing the blood-brain barrier so that they can be used by the brain. In other words, one simple and highly effective way of boosting your circulating SAMe levels is by taking SAMe supplements.

How does SAMe boost the brain population of these neurotransmitters?

SAMe does its work in three basic and rather different ways: by regulating the breakdown of the neurotransmitters, by speeding production of the receptor molecules the neurotransmitters attach themselves to, and by making existing receptor molecules more responsive. The methylation set in action by SAMe is the key factor in each one of these ways.

Protein methylation is necessary for cellular health—both cell growth and cell repair—and that includes the cells of the brain. Thus, protein methylation keeps neurotransmitters healthy, which keeps them from dying off prematurely. Protein methylation also activates cell membrane receptors, ensuring that the transfer of neurotransmitters is quick, smooth, and efficient, another way of keeping the neurotransmitters from ending up as waste products. Looking at it from the other direction, inadequate protein methylation results in slowed down organ processes; in the case of the brain, one such result is clinical depression.

DNA methylation is necessary for activating genes which, in turn, are necessary for regulating cell growth, repair, and reproduction. In the brain, DNA methylation regulates these processes in brain cells and in neurotransmitters. Without adequate DNA methylation, these cells are "poorly managed," resulting in abnormal cell growth (including tumors), inefficient cell repair, and sluggish cell reproduction. Once again, in the brain this result may be experienced as depression.

Finally, there is phospholipid methylation. When the membranes of nerve cells are incapable of accepting such neurotransmitters as serotonin or dopamine, depression is sure to follow. But SAMe appears to stimulate the production of phospholipids, which in turn keep nerve membranes in tip-top condition, making them more able to accept these critical, mood-affecting neurotransmitters.

Please take note—SAMe provides (at least) three different ways to boost the population of these critical antidepressant neurotransmitters! That's two more ways than most of the prescription antidepressants offer. This fact, in itself, does not guarantee anything in terms of SAMe's potency as an antidepressant. But it does account for SAMe's apparent efficacy for a broad group of depression sufferers. If one way of boosting the brain population of neurotransmitters is not effective for a particular individual, one or both of the other two ways may be effective. This is why some doctors refer to SAMe as a "broad spectrum" antidepressant. It appears to work for a greater number of different people than other known antidepressants.

Does SAMe treat depression in any ways besides boosting the brain population of neurotransmitters?

Yes. First, by regulating stress hormones such as adrenaline, SAMe helps control anxiety. And, as we have observed in our discussions of other products that help control anxiety disorders—melatonin, kava-kava, valerian root, L-tryptophan, and 5-HTP—curbing anxiety often has the indirect effect of reducing depression. In a nutshell: People with anxiety disorders feel that they have lost control of their lives and this, in turn, causes them to experience depression; when curing anxiety helps a person regain a sense of control of her life, the cause for that depression is removed.

Second, as we will see later on, SAMe may play a crucial role in preventing and treating Parkinson's disease and Alzheimer's disease, two seriously debilitating diseases that particularly strike older people. In this way, SAMe can play an indirect but important role in mitigating against age-related and chronic-illness related depression.

The large number and variety of functions that SAMe molecules perform in the body leads most scientists to believe that there may be many other ways that SAMe controls depression—ways that have not been discovered.

Are there ways other than taking SAMe supplements for boosting the amount of SAMe circulating in our brains?

Yes, via diet and other supplements.

As the amino acid methionine is critical for our natural internal production of SAMe, a diet that is rich in this amino acid helps ensure our natural production of the SAMe molecule. That means lots of fish, meat, and dairy products; unfortunately, the last two items on this list, when eaten in excess, are associated with heart disease, strokes, and some cancers. Further, such a diet alone does not guarantee elevated SAMe production; it can only mitigate against possible underproduction due to a diet deficient in methionine.

Our internal production of SAMe is also dependent on certain nutrients, particularly vitamin B_{12} and folic acid. But again, megadosing these nutrients is a far from dependable or efficient way to boost natural SAMe production. It is impossible to know just how much of these nutrients would go toward the synthesis of SAMe because so much is determined by the individual's genetic predisposition to make this conversion.

So yes, there are other ways for boosting our natural production of SAMe, but so far, none of these are considered dependable.

How long does it take to feel the first antidepressant effects of SAMe?

Only one to three weeks at the recommended initial dosage. (More about the recommended dosage later.) But a significant number of people report some relief of depression during the first week of taking the supplement. In other words, SAMe shows effects faster than any of the prescription antidepressants. Just why this is so is not completely clear. However, most scientists believe that SAMe's remarkable speed in relieving depression is a result of its "triple-threat" action of providing three different ways of boosting the population of critical antidepressant neurotransmitters.

Two statistically sound studies demonstrated just how fast the response rate with SAMe is compared to other antidepressants. One of these studies, involving almost 200 subjects, showed significant relief of depressive symptoms in 7 to 14 days, as compared to a response rate of 21 days for the fastest-acting prescription antidepressants, and 25-plus days for St. John's wort.

Another response-rate study compared subjects taking SAMe plus the tricyclic antidepressant imipramine with subjects taking only imipramine. Symptoms of depression decreased almost 1.5 times faster on the combined dosage as with the imipramine alone. (More about combining SAMe with other antidepressants later in this chapter.)

The fact that response rate to SAMe is so fast is critically important in the personal decision of whether or not to try SAMe for depression: You only have to try it for a maximum of three weeks to know whether it works for you.

What are the reported side effects of SAMe?

Just about all of the common side effects of SAMe fall into the category of *welcome* side effects. For starters, it clearly helps relieve the symptoms of osteoarthritis (and a surprising number of people will only realize that they were experiencing some arthritic pain and/or stiffness when, as a result of taking SAMe, these symptoms go away).

SAMe also has the side effect of reducing symptoms of fibromyalgia and some liver ailments. And there is some indication that SAMe may also have the side effect of preventing or delaying onset of Parkinson's disease and Alzheimer's disease. But more about all of these happy side effects in subsequent sections of this book.

The important point is that SAMe produces virtually no unwelcome side effects. A very small number of people have reported mild stomach upset from taking the supplement; and an even smaller number have reported brief manic episodes as a result of taking SAMe (these cases were later identified as patients suffering from bipolar disorder as compared to unipolar depression). But that's it. In other words, unlike the major prescription antidepressants, SAMe does not produce decreased sexual drive, nausea, headache, insomnia, anxiety, fatigue and/or excessive sleeping, dry mouth, diarrhea, dizziness, muscle pain, sore throat, night sweats, tremors, itching, visual disorders, or palpitations.

Every one of the above symptoms is a reported side effect of some statistically significant segment of the population taking prescription antidepressants. And for that reason alone, SAMe is preferrable to these drugs.

This is another fact that is critically important in the personal decision of whether or not to try SAMe for depression: If you try SAMe to see whether it works for you, you are running no risks of side effects.

One caveat: as with any first-time use of a new drug, for the first week do not drive or use heavy machinery within the first few hours of taking SAMe on the very remote chance that it may slow down your reflexes.

So it is safe to take SAMe?

Yes. Not only are there no statistically significant unwelcome side effects from taking SAMe, but there are no statistically significant cases of illness or mortality associated with taking SAMe.

Remember, although SAMe is not a prescription drug in the United States and therefore has not undergone the rigorous FDA-mandated testing for safety required of prescription drugs in this country, SAMe *is* a prescription drug in Germany, Italy, and Spain, all countries with high, government-monitored safety standards. If SAMe were not absolutely safe, it would not be permitted to be prescribed or sold in those countries.

For the overall population of depressives, how effective is SAMe as a treatment?

Very. According to controlled studies, over 70% of depressed patients respond to SAMe. This is the same percentage—or slightly more—that responds to the current prescription antidepressants of choice in the United States.

Does SAMe work for moderate and severe depression as well as for mild depression?

Yes. And whereas the other over-the-counter antidepressants only appear to be consistently effective for mild depression, SAMe has an outstanding cure rate in people suffering from severe depression.

One recent study conducted at the University of California at Irvine compared similar populations of severely depressed persons who were given either a standard dosage of SAMe or a standard dosage of the popular prescription tricyclic desipramine. The SAMe group had a higher cure rate (62%) than the desipramine group (50%).

Of course, like the prescription antidepressants, SAMe's cure rate is somewhat higher for mild and moderate depression than for severe depression.

Does SAMe work for manic depression (bipolar disorder)?

No, at least not alone. Just as the normal arsenal of prescription antidepressants (tricyclics, SSRIs, and MAO inhibitors) are not effective as the sole medication for biopolar disorder, neither is SAMe.

Also, as noted above, someone suffering from bipolar disorder may experience manic episodes if he takes SAMe.

Just how thoroughly has SAMe been tested as an antidepressant?

Better by far than most over-the-counter antidepressants, but not as thoroughly as the FDA would require if SAMe were a prescription drug.

To date, most of the studies of SAMe have been done in European countries where SAMe has been prescribed as an antidepressant for over 25 years. Let's look at these first.

By and large, the European tests were self-reporting studies involving relatively small groups of subjects over short periods of time. (The same can be said of the great majority of studies of prescription antidepressants in the United States; for example, to date there are no studies of the long-term effects of taking Prozac.) Because the samples in each of these studies is relatively small, they become statistically significant only when they are viewed collectively in meta-analyses—that is, analyses that combine data in related studies. In the studies combined for analysis here, a total of over 1,000 subjects were tested.

A word about self-reporting: Subjects in such tests record their subjective assessment of their mood on a regular (usually, daily) basis—on days *before* taking the antidepressant or placebo and on days *after* starting to take the antidepressant or placebo. Self-reporting is usually done on a standarized scale called the Hamilton Depression Scale (HAM-D). The responses are quantified in terms of identifiable elements of depression and scored as follows: If 25% to 49% of these elements are resolved, the response to treatment is deemed a "partial response"; if 50% or more are resolved, the response to treatment is deemed a "full response."

So what are the results of these meta-analyses?

Of six studies comparing SAMe with a placebo (a benign "sugar pill" that the testee is led to believe actually may be a drug), five of the studies showed a partial response rate of 70% for those taking SAMe, compared to a partial response rate of 30% for those taking placebos. The "full response" rate was 38% for SAMe as compared to 22% for the placebo. (Although you may be surprised and impressed by the high percentage of "cures" for a placebo, such an effect is not at all unusual in the short term—but short term is usually as long as the "placebo effect" lasts.) Probably the most significant aspect of the SAMe/placebo tests is that SAMe comes out stronger on these tests than prescription antidepressants do on prescription antidepressants/placebo tests.

The studies directly comparing the effects of SAMe with prescription antidepressants are even more impressive except for the fact that the only prescription antidepressants used in such studies to date are the tricyclics (amitriptyline, chlorimipramine, imipramine, and desipramine). That means that as of this time we do not have sufficient data comparing SAMe with the more popularly prescribed SSRIs, including Prozac. (However, what we *do* know is the response rates for the tricyclics and the SSRIs are roughly the same, and that in itself suggests that the SAMe/ SSRI relative response rates would be similar.)

That said, consider the results of this meta-analysis: "Partial response" rates of depressives taking standard doses of SAMe was 92% as compared to 85% for the tricyclics. That is a tremendously significant number for both groups. "Full response" rates were similarly high: 61% for depressives taking standard doses of SAMe and 59% for the tricyclics! And looking at the individual studies that were included in the meta-analysis, we see a marked uniformity of results from study to study.

There has been some testing of SAMe as an antidepressant in the United States, but these tests were also with relatively small test groups by FDA standards. Nonetheless, once again the results uniformly pointed to SAMe's efficacy with all types of depression without unwelcome side effects.

One of these tests at Harvard/Massachusetts General Hospital's Depression Research Center is particularly noteworthy because it included a significant number of patients (9 out of the 20 tested) who had been classified as "treatment resistant." That means that these nine patients had not responded to any other antidepressant medication or to psychological treatment. Put another way, some of these could easily end up as candidates for the depression treatments of last resort, including electroshock therapy. Taking oral doses of SAMe for six weeks, two of these nine showed full response—impressive numbers for patients who never before responded to any other treatment. Of the other (non-treatment-resistant) 11 patients, 7 manifested a full response and two showed partial response—again, highly impressive numbers.

The other most comprehensive American study to date was at the University of California at Irvine, the same university where earlier tests had demonstrated SAMe's effectiveness with severe depression (see above). This study compared response rates to SAMe with those to tricyclics, once more demonstrating that SAMe can more than hold its own against these popular prescription antidepressants. What is particularly interesting about this study is that *all* the patients were tested for SAMe circulating in their blood plasma, regardless of whether they had taken SAMe supplements or a tricyclic antidepressant. Of those showing complete recovery from depression from either medication, *all* showed elevated SAMe levels. In other words, whatever caused the increased concentration of SAMe in these patients' blood plasma, this increase was a prime indicator of full recovery from depression.

To sum up, the evidence is strong that SAMe supplements are as good or better than tricyclics at treating depressions of all kinds—including severe depression—with far fewer side effects. At this point, however, no significant studies have been made comparing SAMe with the SSRIs, including Prozac, and none of the studies have been done with sufficient numbers of patients to qualify for FDA testing standards.

Are you saying that the experimental evidence that SAMe works for depression is not conclusive yet?

Technically, yes: There is not enough rigorous evidence to say unequivocally by FDA standards that SAMe works for depression. But still, there is a great deal of high-grade evidence that shows that it does. And there is more than enough evidence to demonstrate that SAMe is safe and without significant side effects—which is quite a bit more than one can say about any of the prescription antidepressants.

In summation, if you are suffering from depression of any kind, it makes perfect sense to try SAMe as the treatment of first resort because:

1. There is no risk either in terms of safety or unwanted side effects.
2. The response rate is so fast that you will know within three weeks at most whether or not this medication works for you.
3. FDA standards notwithstanding, there is a

preponderance of evidence that SAMe is highly effective for treating all types of depression.

How is SAMe used in conjunction with other anti-depressants?

In Europe, SAMe is commonly used in conjunction with prescription antidepressants for three reasons:

First, the combination of SAMe and a tricyclic is often used with new patients to jump-start the response. Together, SAMe and tricyclics have been demonstrated to get quicker partial and full responses than tricyclics alone. For that matter, SAMe alone has been demonstrated to get quicker responses than tricyclics alone, but many doctors prefer to include tricyclics in their treatment for a variety of reasons ranging from professional habit to because the tricyclics have a proven record of long-term efficacy.

Second the combination of SAMe and a tricyclic is sometimes used so that the dosage of the tricyclic can be reduced in order to minimize the side effects of this prescription antidepressant. Again, one might say that the most dependable way to minimize side effects is to use SAMe alone, but most M.D.s are not ready for that daring step.

And third, the combination of SAMe and a tricyclic is sometimes used as a "fail safe" treatment, as in, "If the one does not work, the other may." Obviously, this is not good science—perhaps one or the other treatment would work for a particular individual *on its own* and this way no one will ever know if that is true. But for a patient who finally experiences relief from depression, questions of "good science" are usually of little interest; she is perfectly willing to take a combination of medications one of which may not have any effect as long as she feels better.

There is a fourth reason for taking both SAMe and a prescription antidepressant that may apply to some readers of this book: If you are currently taking a prescription antidepressant and want to try switching to SAMe, you may want to make this switch gradually. This technique is used by many practicing psychiatrists but should only be tried under the supervision of a psychiatrist or psychopharmacologist.

So there is no danger in adding SAMe to my current antidepressant regime?

The only possible danger is if you are taking an MAO inhibitor (as we have seen, MAO inhibitors "inhibit" the use of scores of foodstuffs and medications). But otherwise there is absolutely no evidence to suggest that adding a dosage of SAMe to your current dosage of a prescription antidepressant causes any harm or unwelcome side effects—and this includes the SSRIs (Prozac). In fact, the most commonly reported "side effect" (and these are only anecdotal reports) of adding SAMe to prescription antidepressants is that the patient feels even better—happier, more energetic, optimistic, and so on. In fact, some psychiatrists and psychologists recommend a combination of SAMe and St. John's wort for patients who find that either of these preparations alone is insufficient to deal with their depression.

How and how much SAMe should I take to treat my depression?

SAMe should be taken on an empty stomach, ideally a half hour or more before meals. Also, it is best to take SAMe at regular intervals two or three times a day, rather than all at once.

As to amount, there are two basic schools of thought on this one: The first school says, take a minimum dosage for a three-week trial period and then increase the dosage as indicated; the second school says, take a maximum dosage for a three-week trial period and then decrease the dosage as indicated.

The first school obviously presents the conservative route to take, even though there are no known risks of overdosing on SAMe. As well as being financially conservative, this approach is therapeutically careful because it predisposes the patient to take the minimum dose necessary to feel acceptably better. In other words, once the patient has reached the dosage point where he feels his depression is sufficiently reduced/treated/controlled, he stops increasing his dosage—even though he does not know whether or not he could feel even better at a higher dose.

To go the conservative route, start with a daily dosage of 400 mg (two doses of 200 mg). Take the supplement on an empty stomach at least one half hour before a meal. Because SAMe-induced methylation will not work with low levels of vitamin B_{12} or folic acid, a 1 mg supplement of each of these is recommended in conjunction with SAMe.

If after 21 days you do not feel that your depression has been sufficiently reduced, add another 400 mg daily dose of SAMe to be taken on an empty stomach at a different time of day, for a total of 800 mg per day (four doses of 200 mg). If after another 14 days, you do not feel that your depression has been sufficiently reduced, add another 400 mg daily dose as above for a total of 1,200 mg per day (three doses of 400 mg). And if after another 14 days, you still do not feel that your depression has been sufficiently reduced, add yet another 400 mg daily dose for a total of 1,600 mg per day (four doses of 400 mg). After another two weeks, if you still do not feel significant relief from your depression, SAMe is not the treatment for you.

The other method of dosage is sometimes known as the "fast-action" or "jump-start" approach because at the end of the first 21 days if you do not feel relief from your depression, you know that SAMe is not the treatment for you, end of story. But looking at it the other way, if at the end of those first 21 days you *do* experience relief from your depression (and for the great majority this will be the case), you know that SAMe works for you—the only question is how much you should take.

There is one reason that some psychiatrists recommend going the "fast-action" route. The fact of the matter is that when you suffer from depression you do not feel much hope about anything—including the hope of ever feeling better. This makes you both cynical and impatient—so cynical and impatient that if you do not feel significantly better after two or three weeks of taking any dosage, small or large, of any medication, you are quite likely to call it quits right then and there.

Furthermore, the fast-action route is not necessarily any less economical than the conservative route: Yes, your initial dosage of SAMe is higher and therefore more expensive; but if it takes you 6, 9, 12, or even 16 weeks to reach the dosage that relieves your depression, you will have paid for several weeks of dosage without the effect you are paying for. Also, the fast action approach is not any riskier than the conservative approach in terms of safety or side effects for the simple reason that there are no known risks at any level of dosage.

One argument against the fast-action approach is worth considering, although ultimately this is more an argument about values than about what is better medicine. Just as the conservative approach predisposes the patient to take the minimum dose necessary to feel acceptably better, the fast-action approach predisposes the patient to take the maximum dose that she feels comfortable with. In other words, if at the maximum dose (1,600 mg) the patient feels just wonderful—better than she ever expected to feel—she will probably stop right there and never decrease her dosage—even though she does not know whether or not she would feel sufficiently "undepressed" at a lower dose.

Here's the fast-action regime: Start with a daily dosage of 1,600 mg SAMe, taken in four separate 400 mg doses, each taken on an empty stomach at least one half hour before a meal. Again, a 1 mg daily dose of vitamin B_{12} or of folic acid is recommended along with the SAMe.

If after 21 days, you do not feel that your depression has been sufficiently reduced, call it quits—and, if you have never sought medical/psychiatric help before, do so now. But if after 21 days you do feel your depression has been sufficiently reduced and you wish to take the minimum dosage necessary to continue feeling this way, subtract 400 mg from your daily dose of SAMe for a new total of 1,200 mg per day (three doses of 400 mg). If after 14 days at this dosage, you do not feel as good as you did at 1,600 mg and you want to continue to feel the way you did at 1,600 mg, immediately go back to that dosage and stay there. But if after 14 days at the 1,200 mg dosage you either feel the same as you did at 1,600 mg or not quite as good but "sufficiently" better (your personal judgment call), either stay there or go to the next step, which is to reduce dosage by another 400 mg for a daily total of 800 mg (two doses of 400 mg). Repeat as desired down to 400 mg per day.

How do I know for sure if I feel better, worse, or the same at different levels of dosage?

Obviously, there is no objective way of measuring these things. And if you are not seeing a therapist in conjunction with your SAMe therapy, you cannot get a professional's evaluation of your symptoms. (Asking your spouse or friends to evaluate your mood is definitely a bad idea for obvious reasons.) If you want to, you can obtain a copy of the Hamilton Depression Scale (HAM-D) from a psychology text and administer it to yourself daily.

But the best way I know for keeping a running record of your mood is by keeping a "mood diary," making entries at the same time or times each and every day. I recommend one entry at lunchtime—a convenient time for most working people and a time of day when our mood is usually at a relatively high point. And I recommend a second entry at around 4:00, when many people, especially depressives, experience their lowest mood of the day.

Ask yourself, "How do I feel?" and write down your spontaneous response. Then break the question down in parts:

- "Do I feel empty today or not?"
- "Do I look at the world and at the people around me negatively or somewhat positively today?"
- "Do I feel sad or kind of happy today?"

- "Do I feel worthless or kind of valuable in some ways today?"
- "Do I feel guilty or not so guilty today?"
- "Do I feel tense and/or nervous today or not so?"
- "Do I feel pessimistic or hopeful today?"
- "Do I feel apathetic or enthusiastic today?"
- "Do I feel lonely or connected to people today?"
- "Do I have a problem concentrating today?"
- "Do I have a problem making decisions today?"
- "Do I feel sluggish today?"
- "Did I have trouble sleeping last night?"

If you are so moved, jot down short first-person narratives of events and personal interactions in your day to illustrate and expand your answers to these questions. And if you want to attempt to quantify your moods, assign a scale of, say, 1 to 10 as responses to each answer. Do not consult previous days' responses until you have reached the end of the evaluation period (14 or 21 days). At that time, read over all your responses carefully and determine for yourself if your mood appears to have consistently improved.

If SAMe relieves my depression, should I take it for the rest of my life?

It depends on the individual and the philosophy of the psychiatrist. In most cases, depression is not like a cold or food poisoning in that once it is cured, you no longer have to treat it. The source of your depression—whether physical or psychological or some ineffable combination of the two—usually remains buried somewhere inside you and may be triggered at any time. Taking SAMe after your depression is gone is a prophylactic measure—it prevents the depression from returning. And being confident that your depression will not return is a significant part of the cure itself because the fear of becoming depressed in the future exerts a powerfully limiting force on us in the present. It narrows the options of feelings and actions that we feel are available to us.

On the other hand, the fact remains that the longer we go without becoming depressed, the less likely we are to ever get depressed again. And so, after some period of time—a year or two or three—we may wish to see if we can do without SAMe. If depression eventually comes back, we can always return to the SAMe treatment.

Isn't that a better idea—rather than using SAMe as a crutch for the rest of my life?

I am afraid the old "crutch" argument doesn't carry much weight for me. Is it a crutch to wear glasses for the rest of your life? Or to take blood pressure pills for the rest of your life? For some reason, we demand of ourselves more self-reliance on mental health issues than we demand of ourselves on so-called strictly physical issues like our eyesight or blood pressure. Other than the expense, what exactly is so awful or shameful about taking an antidepressant that has no side effects for the rest of your life? Because it means that you cannot rid yourself of your depression on your own? Hey, we already knew that.

Isn't there a danger that SAMe will lose its efficacy after years of taking it?

Unlike some prescription antidepressants, like Prozac, SAMe does not appear to lose its potency after extended use. However, the supplement has not been used long enough in this country for any significant data on its life potency to be available.

How does the cost of SAMe compare with other antidepressants?

The cost of SAMe supplements vary rather widely (see Appendix A, "Buying SAMe"), but a conservative estimate puts the cost of average dosage for treating depression at $75 a month.

That is very expensive compared to other over-the-counter antidepressants like St. John's wort, which may cost as little as $15 a month for treating mild depression. But it is less expensive than virtually all prescription antidepressants like Prozac, which costs on average over $90 a month.

It is important to note, however, that while some health insurance programs cover the cost of prescription antidepressants, hardly any cover the cost of over-the-counter medications, including SAMe. Some insurance programs will make an exception to this rule if your doctor in effect "prescribes" the over-the-counter medication in the form of a letter that can be sent to your insurance company.

Is it possible to overdose on SAMe?

No instances of serious effects at high doses have been reported.

Are there any drug interactions with SAMe that I should be aware of?

Only the one that I mentioned, the MAO inhibitor antidepressants. (SAMe is just one of a 10-page list of foods and medications that should not be taken with this drug.)

Is it dangerous to drink alcohol while taking SAMe?

No, and this sets it apart from the prescription antidepressants. Nonetheless, alcohol is a depressant in its own right, so it is never advised for people prone to depression. (Unsurprisingly, some studies show that people who take SAMe for depression find it easier to withdraw from excessive alcohol use and/or dependancy. The reason, many believe, is fairly simple: Often people either consciously or unconsciously drink to "feel no pain"; with SAMe, the "pain" is gone already.)

Can SAMe be used in conjunction with psychotherapy?

Yes. And for many people this is the most beneficial, life-enriching route to take because it combines the best of both worlds of treatment: the relief of the pain and symptoms of depression without unwelcome side effects plus a personal context for understanding yourself as a person recovering from depression who now has a whole new set of life options ahead of you.

First, let's consider the results of successfully taking SAMe (or any other antidepressant) alone—that is, not in conjunction with any kind of psychotherapy. The pain of depression rather quickly recedes, and vanishing with it are most or all of depression's accompanying feelings—feelings of worthlessness, chronic hopelessness and irrational guilt. Also gone are most or all of depression's most common symptoms—insomnia, fatigue, psychomotor disorders, eating disorders, the inability to concentrate, and the inability to make decisions. Fabulous! You feel like a new person!

But that may turn out to be a bit of a problem. Who exactly is this new person? What does he want? Can you trust your new self?

At first, of course, we are so thrillingly relieved of

the pain and symptoms of depression that such questions may seem unimportant to us, even trivial. Who cares? The pain is gone—that's all that matters! Yet, as time goes on and we try to make sense of our new "self," such questions begin to matter very much indeed.

"I know it sounds strange, but I felt kind of clumsy in my new, undepressed incarnation," one person reported after her three-week full recovery from chronic depression using SAMe. "I have heard of people feeling weird after plastic surgery, like they suddenly found themselves in somebody else's body. Well, I felt like I suddenly found myself in somebody else's nervous system! I didn't recognize my feelings. I didn't know how to act with them."

Such reactions are not uncommon. Some people feel so disoriented by their new depression-free selves that they actually start missing their old depressed selves. "Look, I'd been depressed for pretty much my whole adult life," another recovered depressive reported. "I had a whole set of habits that went with the depressed me and those habits didn't make any sense anymore. So what was I going to do— invent a whole new self to go with this undepressed person? At times, it seemed easier to just go back to my old familiar ways—you know, stop taking the SAMe so I wouldn't have the strain of reinventing myself. I actually had a kind of nostalgia for my depression."

And another person who suddenly found herself

free of the feelings and symptoms of depression after taking SAMe for only one week said simply, "It was like I was all dressed up but had no place to go!"

Not only do the old habits of the depressed self need to be adjusted for the new, depression-free self, but the old relationships of the depressed self need to be adjusted too. This can get extremely sticky because it means that other people in your life have to make adjustments too—adjustments that they may be reluctant to make.

"When I was depressed all the time, I had to call my parents at least three times a week or I'd start to feel sick with guilt," one woman in her early thirties reported. "Well, once the depression was gone, so was the guilt, and I realized that I really only wanted to phone my parents when I felt like it, not when I felt guilty about it. So that's what I did. Well, my mother went ballistic! She was pushing every guilt button she could think of to get me back 'on track.' She *wanted* me to be her guilty little girl again. I can't tell you how sad that made me—not depressed, just genuinely sad. I realized that my mother's love was really for this depressed, guilty person—not the happy, independent person I had become."

It becomes quite clear how psychotherapy can benefit a person who is being successfully medicated for depression. Psychotherapy can help the recovered depressive make adjustments to her new self, help her become comfortable in her new "skin."

"It's a little like helping a person adjust to a new culture with different customs and different ways of interacting," one psychotherapist told me. "And often the first step is convincing the patient that these adjustments are worth the trouble, that they offer a much more gratifying life than simply giving up [the medication] and going back to their old ways."

Psychotherapy can also be crucial in helping a recovered depressive adjust to the changing dynamics in his relationships. Parents, spouses, lovers, friends, and even coworkers may present the new, undepressed person with all kinds of resistance to his change. Consciously or unconsciously, flagrantly or subtly, they may want the old, "dependably depressed" you back again. And it may be difficult to disappoint them. It may also be difficult to refrain from giving them a piece of your mind in your new, less intimidated, and more confident mode. Having an experienced psychologist to talk with about these relationships can make the transition a great deal easier for everyone concerned.

There is another way in which psychotherapy can prove quite valuable to someone who has been successfully treated for depression with SAMe, and that way is the traditional role of psychotherapy: helping you understand who you are and how you got that way. The fact is that it is far easier to reach this kind of self-understanding after you are freed from depression than before because you are no longer terrified by the truth, no longer bridled by how you think facing the truth will make you feel. In fact, once you are free of the constraints of depression, you may find yourself hungering for the truth about your life history and personal relationships. In short, things get reversed: Instead of psychotherapy being used to relieve you of depression, being relieved of depression allows you to dive deeply in psychotherapy.

And what is the value in understanding who you are and how you got that way?

That is one of those irreducible questions. You either feel there is fundamental value in this kind of knowledge or you do not. One of those who strongly advocated this fundamental value was the philosopher Socrates, who put it rather bluntly when he said, "The unexamined life is not worth living."

But once you are free of your depression, can't you figure out all these things on your own?

Yes and no. You certainly are in a better position to make personal adjustments and understand yourself on your own than you were when you were suffering from depression. And although there is no substitute for deeply probing psychotherapy, there certainly are ways you can do much of this work on your own.

One time-honored way is to "talk to yourself" by regularly keeping a diary. In the diary, you can experiment with this new self who is emerging from the old. Ask yourself:

- What did you used to be afraid of that you are not afraid of anymore?
- Now that you no longer have these fears, what new options are out there for you?
- What did you used to feel guilty about that you no longer feel guilty about?
- Now that you no longer feel this guilt, what new options are out there for you?
- What old habits are not necessary any more and how should I replace them?
- What old relationships are not working anymore and what should I do about them now?
- What experiences led me to become the person I am? Is this the person I want to be?

The sad fact is that most of us only keep diaries for solace when we are depressed. So keeping a diary when we are finally free of depression is an entirely new experience. It is not only an experience of self-discovery, but an experience in discovering the person you can now become.

PART II

SAMe and Arthritis

EIGHT

Arthritis: What Is It and Who Gets It?

What is arthritis?

Arthritis is a group of diseases that destroy cartilage in the joints and results in inflammation of the joints. It is painful—often quite painful—and can severely limit motion and activity. In its most common form, osteoarthritis, it affects 68% of the population over the age of 65 (as compared to 2% for people 45 and under) and is the third most common disease seen by family doctors.

In order to understand how arthritis does its damage, we need to know a bit about cartilage. Cartilage is an integral part of the skeleton, a specialized fibrous connective tissue. Sometimes known as gristle, it is a pearly, elastic substance attached to bone surfaces and covering the ends of the bones. As a kind of flexible scaffolding, it fastens one bone to another while allowing independent movement of the bones connected at the joint. Cartilage also serves as a gasket or lining between bones at the joint, providing a smooth surface for the bones to slide against. In this function, it keeps the bones from rubbing and scraping against one another, rather like the way the lining of an automobile brake keeps the brake shoe and the wheel from rubbing and scraping against one another.

Therefore when cartilage wears away, the roughened surface of the bone is exposed, the bones grind against one another, and the pain, stiffness, immobility of arthritis follows. In extreme cases of arthritis, the very center of the bone wears away, leaving a bony ridge around the edges. This ridge can severely limit movement of the joint.

Osteoarthritis is the *only* type of arthritis that responds to treatment with SAMe, so that is the specific disease we will be focusing on here. But it is important to know some of the basics about the other forms of arthritis so that confusion does not result in mistaken treatment.

Besides osteoarthritis, there is rheumatoid arthritis, septic arthritis, and a form of arthritis known as gout.

RHEUMATOID ARTHRITIS

Unlike osteoarthritis, rheumatoid arthritis usually begins early, between the ages of 20 and 40. It strikes more women than men, in a ratio of 2:1. And it can strike *any* of our joints, not just those that endure the most daily wear and tear.

The most common symptoms of rheumatoid arthritis include generalized fever, loss of appetite, weight loss, and fatigue—none of which are symptoms of osteoarthritis. Another symptom that often appears in rheumatoid arthritis but rarely occurs in osteoarthritis is redness of the soft tissue surrounding the affected joints.

Rheumatoid arthritis usually starts in the small joints of the hands and feet, then progresses to the larger joints. In acute rheumatoid arthritis, pain tends to migrate from one joint to another; also in acute rheumatoid arthritis, nodules develop under the skin at the sites of bony prominences. Known complications include pericarditis, pleurisy, and blood vessel inflammation.

Symptoms that rheumatoid arthritis have in common with osteoarthritis include stiff, sore joints, usually in the fingers, wrists, knees, ankles, and toes, and swelling and tenderness in the soft tissue surrounding the affected joints. Chronic rheumatoid arthritis often results in deformity in joint areas and in permanent immobility of joints.

The cause of rheumatoid arthritis is unknown. But there are some indications that it has a hereditary component—it clearly runs in families. There are also indications that it is related to some immune system disorders, although no cause and effect has yet been established. Some doctors believe that rheumatoid arthritis is caused by low-grade infections; others believe psychological stress and/or hormone imbalance are at the root of the disease.

The disease can suddenly disappear—burn out completely without any long-term effects. But it can also just as suddenly and unexpectedly reappear and continue with progressive joint inflammation and deformity.

There is no definitive cure for rheumatoid arthritis. Medical treatment addresses the main symptom of the disease, the inflammation, with analgesic pain relievers like aspirin, and with nonsteroidal anti-inflammatories like ibuprofen (more about both of these when we discuss osteoarthritis). Some doctors treat rheumatoid arthritis with gold salts, but there are no conclusive tests showing that this treatment works. Most doctors recommend applying heat to the affected areas and following carefully regulated programs of alternating rest and therapeutic exercise.

In advanced cases, steroids such as cortisone are often used to address a single joint that is extremely inflamed and/or swollen. Some doctors treat the disease with Cloprednol, a hormone product that works like steroids but with fewer side effects; currently, Cloprednol is only available in Mexico.

Surgery is also used in advanced cases, both arthroscopic and joint replacement procedures. But again, more about both of these when we discuss osteoarthritis.

There are a number of "alternative" and nutritional treatments for rheumatoid arthritis, including special diets, vitamin supplements, acupuncture, and electrical stimulation. All of these are also used for osteoarthritis and will be discussed in detail later on.

SEPTIC ARTHRITIS

Septic arthritis is an infection of a joint (as compared to just an inflammation) that results from either an injury directly to the joint or an infection that spreads from some other site of the bone or through the blood stream to the joint. The infection can be caused by any type of bacteria, but the usual culprit is either staphylococcus, gonococcus (gonorrhea bacteria), or hemophilus influenza. Septic arthritis is a fairly rare form of arthritis; it strikes men and women equally.

Symptoms include sudden pain, swelling, and redness in the affected joint, fever, chills, generalized weakness, nausea, and loss of appetite. There is a good chance that the joint will temporarily become immobile as a result of the pain and swelling. Septic arthritis can last weeks, depending on treatment.

But unlike other kinds of arthritis, treatment can directly address the cause—the bacterial infection— with antibiotics, usually administered intravenously for up to four or five weeks. With quick treatment, recovery is complete and with no lingering arthritic aftereffects.

GOUT

Gout is an acute inflammation of a joint that is caused by deposits of uric acid crystals. It strikes more men than women in a ratio of 9:1 and usually strikes people over the age of 30. Excessive uric acid may be a result of a hereditary predisposition and/or dehydration, fasting, destruction of body tissue (including from cancer), kidney disease, high alcoholic intake, or high caloric intake. Thus people who are overweight or drink excessively appear to be at particular risk. Like septic arthritis, it is a relatively rare form of arthritis.

The symptoms are *sudden* onset of severe pain, redness, swelling, and tenderness of the joint, often at night. The most common joint affected is the big toe. After inflammation subsides, the skin over the affected joint peels and itches. Gout can lead to the formation of kidney stones and to chronic arthritis.

Basic treatment of gout addresses the cause—the excessive uric acid in the bloodstream—with the drug colchicine, which rapidly reduces the blood levels of uric acid. Still, the pain of gout is so severe that the symptoms also have to be attended to—with pain relievers and heat applied to the joint. High (nonalcoholic) liquid intake will help kidneys eliminate excessive uric acid.

OSTEOARTHRITIS

Most medical texts refer to osteoarthritis as "part of the normal aging process." Indeed, it is a degenerative disease (i.e., caused by deterioration of tissue) affecting more that half of people over 65. The tissue in question is, of course, the cartilage that covers the ends of the bones; when it wears away from prolonged use (65 years is prolonged use), the bones become exposed and begin to grind against one another with typical arthritic results: pain, swelling, stiffness, and immobility.

Both men and women are affected, although when osteoarthritis progresses to the stage of bone loss, postmenopausal women—who are naturally prone to calcium deficiencies—are more affected. Women are also more likely than men to experience osteoarthritis in the distal joints of the fingers.

Generally, the weight-bearing joints are most likely to be affected: knees, hips, lower back, and the base of the spine. Next come the neck, shoulders (front area), fingers and thumb knuckle, and the jaw (the temporomandibular joint, known colloquially as TMJ).

Here's a rundown of the most common symptoms of osteoarthritis, stressing those symptoms that differentiate it from other types of arthritis: stiffness in one or more joints, *usually in the morning or after a long period of inactivity*; enlargement of the affected progressive pain in the affected joints, but with *little or no deformity*; intensified joint pain after extended use, followed by limited motion of the affected joint and a grating sensation upon movement. Note that there is no redness or excessive warmth in the tissue around the affected joint and there is no fever.

So the cause of osteoarthritis is simply the normal breakdown of cartilage tissue as a result of joint stress?

Yes and no. Let's start by focusing on the "no," because it is key to the way SAMe can treat osteoarthritis at the causal (as compared to symptomatic) level.

Recent medical evidence suggests that deterioration of cartilage tissue is only half the osteoarthritis story. The other half is that deteriorated cartilage tissue is not regenerated because the cellular mechanism by which cartilage is manufactured and maintained breaks down. So it is not just that this protective material wears away at the joints; it wears away without ever building back up again the way it used to when our bodies were younger and less stressed.

The cellular mechanism that normally keeps our cartilage ship-shape is similar to the mechanism that keeps our skin ship-shape despite the daily wear and tear of scrapes and bruises and other traumas like temperature changes, dryness, and sunburn. New skin cells are regenerated virtually as fast as old skin cells die. Ditto for cartilage cells when all is working well.

But all does *not* work well when our joints are under prolonged stress. Not only does the cartilage break down, but the key components for the making of cartilage also break down: proteoglycan and collagen. The component proteoglycan has a capacity for holding water, which is fundamental for cartilage's cushioning properties; and the component collagen (yes, the same stuff that women have injected into their lips for the pouty look) is the firm yet flexible tissue that permits cartilage to both hold bones together and let them flex at the joints. Both proteoglycan and collagen are manufactured by the body from a third basic component, cells called chondrocytes—and therein lies the problem. Chondrocytes, like all cells, need glucose for energy—but damage to cartilage has the unfortunate effect of reducing glucose's ability to get to the chondrocytes. So here is the unhappy chain of events: no glucose, no chondrocytes, no proteoglycan and collagen, no new cartilage. It is also a vicious circle: no new cartilage, no glucose reaches the chondrocytes, no new protoglycan and collagen, no new cartilage.

These components and mechanisms for regenerating damaged cartilage become relevant when we examine the effects of the current medications of choice for osteoarthritis. And they become especially relevant when we examine how SAMe treats osteoarthritis by actually helping to rebuild damaged cartilage.

But what causes the breakdown of the cartilage in the first place?

At the systemic/chemical level, there are two competing theories for the cause of cartilage breakdown. Some scientists believe it is a result of free radicals wreaking their havoc on the tissue in question (more about this in Chapter 10). Other scientists believe it is a result of the low levels of critical hormones like testosterone, estrogen, and growth hormone that come about naturally with age. These hormones are crucial for managing the repair of tissue, including cartilage.

But the reigning theory is still that the breakdown of cartilage is the cumulative result of the natural wear and tear of living and moving about. This basically translates into three things: too much body weight, too many repeated identical motions, and major traumas. Let's look at these one at a time.

TOO MUCH BODY WEIGHT

Too much body weight inflicts stress on the joints, causing a breakdown of cartilage. How excessive body weight does this is pretty obvious: You don't need to be a civil engineer to know that if a building designed to bear 150 tons of weight is required to support one and a half times that weight, something has to give. It probably will not give all at once—but day by day the stress of carrying more weight than the structure was built to tolerate will break down the struts and beams and walls that are bearing this weight.

The analogy to the body is simple: If your skeletal and muscular structure is "designed" to support 150 pounds of weight and you build up your mass one and a half times that to 225 pounds, something has to give. And chances are what will give are the weight-bearing joints in your knees, hips, and lower back.

TOO MANY REPEATED MOTIONS

Most repeated (repetitive) motions are work-related. For example, typists or piano players perform identical motions with their fingers and wrists hundreds of times daily, pushing and pulling the cartilage in the joints of their fingers and wrists in identical places over and over again. And while a single such motion does not cause any wear and tear on the cartilage, hundreds of identical motions inflicting a minute amount of stress on an identical stretch of tissue can eventually wear that cartilage right down to the bone. Baseball pitchers wear away the cartilage in their shoulders. Ditch diggers wear away the cartilage in their knees and hips.

MAJOR TRAUMAS OR INJURIES

At the other end of the stress spectrum are traumas that essentially "blast" away so much cartilage in a single hit that the area never recovers. (Remember, once enough cartilage is gone, the mechanism for rebuilding cartilage often is gone too.) Automobile and sports injuries are the usual culprits here. That is why it is not unusual to see a man who was once a "bone crusher" on the football field wincing from the pain of osteoarthritis at a fairly young age. His sports injury has come back to haunt him in the form of arthritis.

Is it worth having medical tests to determine what kind—if any kind—of arthritis you have?

Yes, especially if you are considering SAMe treatment for osteoarthritis and therefore need to know for sure that it is *not* rheumatoid arthritis that you are suffering from (rheumatoid arthritis does not respond to SAMe). Two simple and relatively inexpensive tests can determine if you have rheumatoid arthritis: an erythrocyte sedimentation rate test (ESR) and a rheumatoid arthritis factor blood test (RAF).

Many doctors order several very expensive imaging tests for diagnosing arthritis: magnetic resonance imaging (MRI), CAT scans, and X rays of the affected areas. In most cases, the actual amount of information revealed by these tests that is relevant for treatment does not justify the cost and inconvenience of undergoing them; a good doctor can tell virtually all she needs to know from a physical examination, self-reporting of the patient, and the ESR and RAF. (One exception is if nerve root compression—as in sciatica—is suspected; imaging can confirm or deny such a diagnosis.)

It is always hard to resist when a doctor suggests a particular medical test, such as an MRI. But keep in mind that there is a good chance he is recommending this test because the hospital or clinic with which he is affiliated needs to financially justify owning such expensive hardware by using it as frequently as possible.

NINE

The Most Common Treatments for Osteoarthritis

What treatments do doctors most frequently prescribe for osteoarthritis?

Most often, doctors prescribe medicines that address the basic symptoms of osteoarthritis—the inflammation and pain, and the stiffness and immobility that result from the disease. These include over-the-counter analgesics, such as aspirin and acetaminophen; over-the-counter and prescription nonsteroidal anti-inflammatories (NSAIDs) such as ibuprofen, naproxen, and sulindac (Clinoril); and prescription steroids such as prednisone. All of these medications have a number of extremely unwelcome side effects, including gastritis, stomach ulcers, kidney and liver damage, and in the case of steroids, serious hormonal disorders—in short, side effects that often make the cure as bad, if not worse, than the disease.

In severe and intractable cases of osteoarthritis, surgery is sometimes recommended, either arthroscopic surgery or joint replacement. Like all surgery, both of these procedures entail sizable risks.

And in virtually all cases of osteoarthritis doctors recommend specific changes in diet, lifestyle, and exercise regimes.

Let's start with the analgesics—what are they and how do they work?

ASPIRIN

Aspirin has been used to treat arthritis for a hundred years in tablet form and for centuries in its naturally occurring form. It is basically an acid—salicylic acid—that was originally made from the bark of the willow tree and now is synthesized. It is the most popular over-the-counter medication in the United States.

Aspirin works as a pain killer by inhibiting the synthesis and release of hormones called prostaglandins that are responsible for sensitizing nerve receptors to respond to pain messages. In other words, by introducing aspirin, there are fewer prostaglandins floating around, and with fewer prostaglandins floating around, fewer pain messages reach their destination, the end result being less or no pain. For reasons that are less clear, aspirin appears to reduce the inflammation at the joints that contributes to arthritic pain.

In fact, it is surprising how little is known about how this most popular of drugs works its "magic." And that is why it never ceases to amaze me that people who are habitually mistrustful of new over-the-counter medications like SAMe have no problem at all popping aspirins by the handful—a drug that is essentially folkloric in origin, that relatively little is known about, and that has some serious side effects and risks (more about these below).

ACETAMINOPHEN

Acetaminophen, best known by its most popular brand name, Tylenol, is a recently discovered analgesic that is currently the over-the-counter painkiller of choice because it reduces pain without aspirin's most pernicious side effect, stomach problems. On the other hand, as we will see, it has some side effects and risks of its own, and it does not address the inflammation at the root of the arthritic pain, the way aspirin does.

What are the NSAIDs and how do they work?

The nonsteroidal anti-inflammatories are exactly that—medications which are not steroids that reduce inflammation and the pain associated with inflammation. The best-known over-the-counter NSAIDs are ibuprofen (Advil, Motrin) and naproxen; the best-known prescription NSAID is sulindac (Clinoril).

Like aspirin, NSAIDs reduce both pain and inflammation by inhibiting the production and release of prostaglandins. Also like aspirin, NASAIDs produce gastrointestinal distress.

What is the downside of taking the analgesics and NSAIDs?

First, there are the gastrointestinal side effects of both aspirin (but not of other analgesics, such as acetaminophen) and of the NSAIDs, the result of these drugs irritating the stomach lining. In many cases, this is not just a little discomfort—the irritation often evolves into gastritis, bleeding of the stomach lining, and ulcers.

Dosage matters a great deal in this regard. For example, in most cases four aspirin a day does not result in gastritis or bleeding; but on the other hand, four aspirin a day is rarely anywhere near enough to deal with the pain and inflammation of moderate osteoarthritis. So at effective doses, these drugs do present a serious risk of gastrointestinal side effects.

Let me put the seriousness of that risk in numerical perspective: 103,000 Americans each year end up in the hospital as a result of NSAID-induced ulcers—and of those, 16,500 die. So we are not just talking about some merely "annoying" side effect here.

There are, of course, ways to reduce the incidence

and severity of gastrointestinal side effects of taking aspirin or a NSAID. Obviously, taking the offending medications at meals will help. And taking buffered or coated aspirin can help too. Another simple and relatively inexpensive strategy is to take antacids along with the drugs—lots of them. These days, the over-the-counter options for antacids go far beyond Tums and the like: Zantac and Tagamet go a long way in reducing reflux and gastritis and all the gastrointestinal damage that follows from them.

Second, there are the blood-thinning side effects of aspirin and the NSAIDs. In addition to their capacity to inhibit production and release of prostaglandins, these drugs also interfere with platelet production (blood clotting). This, of course, is good news for people who are at risk for heart attacks—taking aspirin and/or NSAIDs reduces the likelihood of producing a clot in a coronary artery, which is the way a heart attack begins. But it is extremely bad news for the large number of people who are at risk for internal bleeding—and high on that list are people who are at such risk because of stomach ulcers. So this is a way in which the side effects gang up with one another to wreak havoc on the body.

Both kidney and liver damage are also possible side effects of NSAIDs and aspirin. In the kidney, the damage results from reduced blood-flow to the organ with outcomes of fluid retention, protein loss in urine, high blood pressure, and, finally, kidney failure. This is a rare side-effect (especially of aspirin), but for people who are prone to kidney problems—like diabetics—it needs to be taken into account when assessing the risk of taking these drugs to treat arthritis.

Liver damage as a result of NSAID or aspirin intake is also a rare side effect, but especially in the case of chronic use of acetaminophen it is well worth noting because the outcome can be hepatitis—including fatal hepatitis. Not unsurprisingly, the risk of liver damage with either of these arthritis drugs is exacerbated by moderate-to-high alcohol intake.

But the most alarming side effect of both aspirin and NSAIDs on patients who are taking them for symptoms of osteoarthritis is that they actually contribute to cartilage deterioration. In other words, these "cures" aggravate the central cause of the disease!

You may recall that the key components for the body's synthesis of cartilage are proteoglycan and collagen, which in turn are manufactured by the body from a third basic component, cells called chondrocytes. Well, it turns out that aspirin and NSAIDs suppress the ability of chondrocytes to make proteoglycan. This, as we've noted before, starts a destructive spiral going: The depletion of proteoglycan leaves the chonodrocytes even more vulnerable to destruction—and on it goes with the end result of damaged cartilage that is now unable to regenerate.

It even gets worse. It turns out that the NSAIDS are even more destructive of cartilage damaged by osteoarthritis than of normal cartilage (the damaged cartilage takes up the NSAIDs more easily than unaffected cartilage does). This goes way beyond the cure being worse than the disease—in this case, the cure exacerbates the disease.

The contrast of aspirin and the NSAIDs with SAMe as a treatment for osteoarthritis becomes especially poignant in this light: Whereas aspirin and the NSAIDs contribute to the further destruction of arthritis-damaged cartilage, SAMe contributes to the regeneration of arthritis-damaged cartilage.

What are the steroids and how do they work?

Steroids are complex molecules that are of basic importance in our bodies' chemistry, particularly in our sex and adrenal hormones. Synthesized and administrated either orally or by injection, steroids are used in the treatment of a variety of disorders, including hormone deficiencies, some allergies, and arthritis. (Steroids are also used, illegally, to build muscle mass in weight-lifters and other athletes.)

If a single joint is severely affected by arthritis of any kind, some doctors will inject the site of the inflammation with one of any number of the synthetic steroids. Relief from the symptoms is often quick and dramatic—the patient goes from extreme pain and immobility to painlessness and full-range use of the affected joint within hours. Unfortunately, the long-term effects can sometimes also be dramatic: patients given synthetic steroids may come down with serious endocrine (hormone) disorders, including one that is, for all intents and purposes, the same as the severely debilitating and disfiguring hormonal disease Cushing's syndrome, which is caused by the adrenal gland's overproduction of the naturally occurring hormone cortisol. However, the long-term effects of taking the steroids cortisone or prednisone *orally* over an extended period of time are more hazardous.

What types of surgery are used for osteoarthritis?

Two types, arthroscopy and joint replacement, both of which offer only short-term relief.

Today, as a result of fiber optics and modern microsurgery, arthroscopy has become a relatively quick and efficient surgical procedure that can be performed on an out-patient basis. Pinpointing the affected joint through tiny punctures, "shaggy" cartilage is shaved away and sucked off, leaving the remaining cartilage smooth. The result is a dramatic reduction in pain and expanded movement in the affected joint. The bad news, however, is that by shaving away cartilage, this lining gets thinner—closer to the bone, as it were, causing one critical aspect of the disease to actually get worse.

Joint replacement surgery is a more complex procedure—longer, more costly, and with all the attendant risks of a general anesthetic. But for both baseball pitchers with rotary-cuff injuries and regular folk with osteoarthritis, joint replacement can offer a new lease on life, especially in terms of movement. Older sufferers who were previously unable to walk due to osteoarthritis in the hips and/or knees are able to hop, skip, and jump after having the old, affected joints replaced with new, synthetic ones. In addition to the risk of this surgery (which is not *that* great), the problem with replaced joints is they generally have a relatively short half-life—they wear out easily, requiring repeat surgery.

Are there any other therapies for reducing the pain and inflammation of osteoarthritis?

Heat—especially as applied to the affected joint—is the time-honored way of reducing both the pain and the inflammation of osteoarthritis. Heat can be applied to specific areas with heating pads, hot water bottles, hot moist towels, or heating lamps. And heat can be applied to the entire body with hot tub baths and paraffin baths. I have heard some people swear by sleeping in a sleeping bag as a way to keep the body extra warm, resulting in a therapeutic sleep. The results of heat therapies are temporary relief of pain, inflammation, and swelling.

Massage therapy also provides relief from both the pain and inflammation of osteoarthritis, especially if you are "in the hands" of a masseur who specializes in arthritis relief. Not only does massage therapy reduce the muscle tension associated with arthritis—and hence the spasms that sufferers often experience around the joint—but massage offers a form of "passive" exercise that helps expand the range of motion by improving flexibility and building muscles that prevent further injuries to the affected areas. In addition to regular Swedish massage, shiatsu and acupressure massage can go a long way in relieving the pain of arthritis. So can the skeletal manipulations of chiropractics and osteopathy, although extreme care is recommended in these therapies; by applying strong and sudden pressure to the joints, the therapist can aggravate the inflammation of the cartilage.

The Asian medicine acupuncture—literally puncturing the skin with very thin needles to stimulate "energy centers" of the body—provide relief for the pain and inflammation of osteoarthritis. Many patients claim that their range of motion was quickly and vastly improved by this ancient therapy. Again, be sure of the qualifications and experience of your practitioner—you don't want an amateur sticking needles in you.

Two other popular forms of therapy address the pain and inflammation of osteoarthritis—so-called "healing" magnets and transcutaneous electrical nerve stimulation (TENS)—but neither has been sufficiently tested to merit an unqualified recommendation.

How do lifestyle and exercise affect osteoarthritis?

In a word: immensely! To begin, weight loss is essential in any program to prevent or slow the progress of osteoarthritis. The reason why this is so should be obvious by now: If you ask your skeletal structure to bear more weight than it is built to bear, something has to give. And one of the first things to give is the cartilage in the weight-bearing joints—particularly the hips and knees. If you are serious about stemming the deterioration wrought by osteoarthritis, bringing your weight down to the absolute minimum ideal weight for your height and gender is a must. And you have to keep it there, because frequent weight fluctuations put an additional strain on your joints. Even with the effective medical intervention that I believe SAMe to be, maintaining low body weight is mandatory.

Next, exercise is essential in any program to prevent or slow the progress of osteoarthritis. Again, the reasons for this should be obvious: First, inactivity causes joints to stiffen and activity keeps them flexible; second, exercise helps maintain low body weight; and third, exercise that leads to building stronger muscles around the affected joint makes that joint more stable and less likely to incur further cartilage-damaging trauma. Like weight loss, exercise should be part of any medical program for treating osteoarthritis.

It is highly important that your exercise program be tailored to your personal condition, arthritic and otherwise. You do not want a program that puts traumatic stress on the very bone and muscle areas you are trying to improve. To this end, I highly recommend either a personal trainer with experience supervising people with osteoarthritis or a physical therapist with the same experience. Such a supervisor will show you how to stretch the muscles in the affected area and how to gradually build up the muscle mass of the critical areas. Further, she will show you how various simple exercises such as walking and swimming (in a warm pool) can be adapted for maximum benefits.

Once again, Eastern philosophies and practices offer some helpful options here in the form of yoga and tai chi, both of which lead you through low-stress, low-impact, slow-motion exercises that stretch and develop muscles and ligaments in affected areas without taxing them.

As fingers and wrists are particularly vulnerable to the deterioration of osteoarthritis (especially for women), exercises that gently exercise the hands are highly recommended. And these days the ubiquitous "hand gyms" you find in drug and health stores are quite helpful in this regard. Studies show that five daily minutes of "hand gym" exercises result in improved finger and wrist strength, range of motion, and useful hand function at the end of only two months.

Like exercise, good posture plays an important role in preventing the stiffness and crippling effects of osteoarthritis. Poor posture can cause body weight to be distributed unevenly, placing more stress on certain joints and resulting in exacerbated arthritic pain. There are professionals who can help you acquire good posture through alignment, breathing, and awareness exercises. The Alexander method, a highly respected form of neo-Reichian therapy that addresses both physical and psychological problems through a series of postural adjustments and exercises, is particularly recommended.

Another lifestyle change that osteoarthritis sufferers obviously need to heed is to cease and desist from those physical practices that put stress on the affected joints. Such stress may be from repetitive motion or from just plain weight strain (like moving pianos). For either a professional pianist or a piano mover, for example, ceasing and desisting from the very activities that support him and/or gives his life meaning would be no small sacrifice. On the other hand, if arthritis progresses far enough, ceasing and desisting from these activities will no longer be a choice—it will be a necessity. Short of stopping such activities altogether, see if you can find different ways to do them—including using mechanical devices such as braces to redistribute the stress and strain. (Also, seek out arthritis-friendly gadgets for daily life—low-strain can openers, pencil grips, etc.) Obviously, no one can make up your mind for you on issues as fundamental as whether or not to abandon some activity in your life; just be sure you are fully informed when you make your decision.

A final recommendation for an arthritis-friendly lifestyle is one that few people have the luxury of choosing: Live in a hot, dry climate. The ubiquitous heat provides ongoing relief from pain, inflammation, and swelling, while the lack of humidity makes this heat more tolerable.

How does diet affect osteoarthritis?

First and foremost, diet affects body weight which, as we have seen, has a pronounced effect on the symptoms and progression of osteoarthritis.

But nutritionists also suggest particular foods and/or supplements to combat osteoarthritis. Among these are foods or supplements that are rich in vitamin C to prevent the capillary walls in the joints from breaking down and causing bleeding, swelling, and pain. There is also some preliminary evidence that supplements of folic acid, vitamin B_{12}, and the minerals calcium, magnesium, and potassium slow the progression of osteoarthritis.

Finally, I should note that many clinics in Europe (especially Sweden) treat osteoarthritis patients with a week-long partial fast of only juices, broths, and teas, followed thereafter with a diet consisting of raw fruits, vegetable salads, yogurt, wheat germ, brewer's yeast, seeds, nuts, vegetable soup, potatoes, prunes, raisins, cottage cheese, and kelp. Some patients swear by it, but no data is available for analyzing its effectiveness in treating either the symptoms or causes of osteoarthritis.

TEN

The SAMe Treatment for Osteoarthritis

How does SAMe treat osteoarthritis?

Like aspirin and the NSAIDs, SAMe treats osteo-arthritis by functioning as a painkiller and an anti-inflammatory, thus reducing or stopping the pain of the arthritis and reducing or stopping the irritation of the cartilage in the affected joints. In this function, SAMe treats the basic symptoms of arthritis.

But there is growing evidence that SAMe goes a major step further than just treating the symptoms of osteoarthritis. Tests now show that SAMe stops the degenerative process of osteoarthritis and actually rebuilds the damaged cartilage that is the prime cause of the disease. In this way, SAMe crosses over from a mere treatment for osteoarthritis to a cure for osteo-arthritis.

How does SAMe achieve this amazing effect?

To answer this question, we'll have to run through a quick review of the chemistry of SAMe and of the chemistry of osteoarthritis, adding a few new relevant points.

THE CHEMISTRY OF SAMe

SAMe is a molecule that is produced in all living cells, including human cells, from a substance called adenosine triphosphate (ATP) and an amino acid called methionine. When our cells produce a sufficient number of SAMe molecules, an essential substance called a methyl group is released, which in turn fuels dozens of biochemical reactions in our bodies. This process, known as methylation, happens over a billion times per second throughout our bodies and is necessary for a variety of fundamentally important life functions ranging from fetal development to brain operation. You will recall that this process of methylation works on, among other things, our DNA, our proteins, and on our cell membranes (phospholipids). Methylation is also critical in the production and regulation of many of our hormones.

Another critical life process that SAMe is intimately involved with is transsulfuration, a process that produces a supremely important substance in our bodies called glutathione. Sometimes called the "master antioxidant," glutathione is at the center of the body defense system that controls those ubiquitous scoundrels in our bodies known as free radicals. (No, free radicals are not a rebellious political action group that takes over our bodies, but for all the damage they do, they might as well be.) Free radicals are the unstable molecules in our bodies and unstable oxygen molecules that are generated by the basic chemical transaction of living: oxidizing calories into energy. When these free radicals accumulate in our systems, the results can be deadly: They can attack our DNA with the possible result of cancer; they can attack the lipids in our blood causing them to turn into the plaque that blocks our arteries and causes heart attacks and strokes; and they can attack brain cells, causing senility.

Thankfully, antioxidants are the natual enemies of free radicals and that is why a diet rich in antioxidants like vitamins C, E, and beta carotene, and L-glutathione is recommended to promote health by protecting against the diseases borne of an overpopulation of free radicals. But better yet is SAMe: It is essential for the transsulfuration process that is the source of the *internal production* of glutathione. Beside functioning as an antioxidant, glutathione also plays an important anti-inflammatory role in our systems.

Now comes the kicker: SAMe is also essential for the production of chondrocytes which in turn are essential for the internal production of proteoglycan—the high-wear, high-production component of cartilage!

THE CHEMISTRY OF OSTEOARTHRITIS

Let's review: Deterioration of cartilage tissue is only half the osteoarthritis story. The other half is that deteriorated cartilage tissue is not regenerated because the cellular mechanism by which cartilage is manufactured and maintained breaks down. So it is not just that this protective material wears away at the joints; it wears away without ever building back up again—the way it used to when our bodies were younger and less stressed.

The cellular mechanism that normally keeps our cartilage ship-shape is similar to the mechanism that keeps our skin ship-shape; new skin cells are regenerated virtually as fast as old skin cells die. Ditto for cartilage cells when all is working well. But all does not work well when our joints are under prolonged stress. Not only does the cartilage break down, but the key components for the making of cartilage also break down: proteoglycan and collagen. The component proteoglycan has a capacity for holding water, which is fundamental for cartilage's cushioning properties; and the component collagen is the firm yet flexible tissue that permits cartilage to both hold bones together and let them to flex at the joints. Both proteoglycan and collagen are manufactured by the body from a third basic component, cells called chondrocytes, and therein lies the problem. Chondrocytes, like all cells, need glucose for energy, but damage to cartilage has the unfortunate effect of reducing glucose's ability to get to the chondrocytes. Thus the degenerative cycle of no glucose, no chondrocytes, no proteoglycan and collagen, no new cartilage.

Now let's look again at some of the suspected systemic causes of osteoarthritis. You will recall that many leading theorists believe that the original cartilage breakdown in osteoarthritis is the result of chronic damage by accumulated free radicals. Other theorists believe that the prime culprit is the natural decline in critical hormones like testosterone, estrogen, and growth hormone—hormones that, among other things, regulate tissue repair in a body.

PUTTING IT ALL TOGETHER

SAMe is critical in production of the master antioxidant glutathione. Inasmuch as the cause of chronic osteoarthritis may be the damage that free radicals do to the cartilage of our joints, and antioxidants knock off free radicals, glutathione is a bonafide treatment for the disease at its source. Add to this that for reasons that are not altogether clear, glutathione functions independently as an anti-inflammatory with results similar to those of aspirin and the NSAIDs, but without their unwelcome side effects. In addition, inasmuch as another cause of osteoarthritis may be the natural deficiences in critical hormones that come with age, and glutathione aids in the production and regulation of these critical hormones, glutathione is once again a bonafide treatment for the disease at its source.

Finally and most importantly, inasmuch as we need chondrocytes to regenerate the fundamental constituents of our cartilage, proteoglycan and collagen, and SAMe is essential for the production of chondrocytes, SAMe is more than a treatment for osteoarthritis—it helps to reverse the course of the disease. For a long time researchers have been searching for a treatment for osteoarthritis that does not waste chondrocytes; in SAMe, not only do we have that, we actually have a substance that stimulates the new production of chondrocytes!

HOW DOES TREATMENT WITH SAMe COMPARE WITH CONVENTIONAL TREATMENTS FOR OSTEOARTHRITIS?

Put bluntly, there is no comparison—SAMe is so far superior to anything else currently being offered by medical science. Of course, the competition is not much to speak of—medical treatment for osteoarthritis is a long-standing embarrassment for the medical/pharmaceutical establishment.

The comparison with the analgesics and NSAIDs is simply this: Both SAMe and the analgesics/NSAIDs reduce pain and inflammation with equal success. But while SAMe has no documented unwelcome side effects of any kind, the analgesics/NSAIDs cause severe gastrointestinal problems including ulcers; cause internal bleeding, which is particularly risky for people with ulcers, and can cause both kidney and liver damage.

And that is the least of it, because while aspirin and the NSAIDs actually suppress the ability of chondrocytes to make that critical piece of cartilage called proteoglycan, SAMe actually promotes the production of chondrocytes—it contributes to the regeneration of arthritis-damaged cartilage. As I said: no comparison!

As to the comparison with steroids, I repeat: SAMe causes no documented unwelcome side effects of any kind. Taking ACT brings a clear risk of endocrine (hormone) disorders, including one that is, for all intents and purposes, the same as the disfiguring hormonal disease Cushing's syndrome, while the long-term effects of taking the steroids cortisone or prednisone orally over an extended period of time are only slightly less debilitating. Add to this the fact that the steroids have no ameliorative effect on the damaged cartilage at the root of osteoarthritis while SAMe contributes to the regeneration of damaged cartilage and one can say once again: no comparison!

When it comes to comparing SAMe with surgical intervention as a treatment for osteoarthritis, we cannot be as definitive in our assessment. Obviously, both arthroscopy and joint replacement entail far greater risks than the virtually risk-free SAMe, but arthroscopy and joint replacement are treatments of last resort for advanced cases of crippling osteoarthritis, and so far SAMe has not been proven as a relief or cure for the disease in this advanced state. However, that said, it would make perfect sense to take SAMe in conjunction with arthroscopy—the surgery would remove "shaggy" and "floating" cartilage while the SAMe would ostensibly promote production of new cartilage to take its place.

How does treatment with SAMe compare with alternative treatments for osteoarthritis?

Here again, it is more helpful to think of "supplementing" than of "comparing."

For example, it makes perfect sense to continue applying heat to affected joints while taking SAMe: The heat will supply short-term relief to pain and inflammation, supplementing SAMe's effects in this regard; the heat may also help to provide an internal environment that abets SAMe's regenerative effects on damaged cartilage. The same can be said of massage therapy and acupuncture.

Is there the same kind of "synergy" between SAMe treatments and lifestyle adjustments for osteoarthritis?

Most definitely. For example, as good as the regenerative powers of SAMe appear to be, they cannot keep pace with the amount of damage to your joints that being overweight causes. So, weight loss—when appropriate—needs to be part of any osteoarthritis treatment, including SAMe treatment. Obviously, the same can be said of exercise, especially inasmuch as exercise leads to stronger muscles around the affected joint, making that joint more stable and less likely to incur further cartilage-damaging trauma. Further, like heat therapy, exercise may help provide an internal environment that abets SAMe's regenerative effects on damaged cartilage. And again, the same can be said of yoga, tai chi, and postural adjustments and exercises. Further, the warnings about physical practices that put stress on the affected joints apply here too: They should be part of any osteoarthritis treatment program, including SAMe treatment.

When it comes to diet (other than for weight reduction) as a supplement to SAMe treatment, there is some evidence that folic acid and vitamin B_{12} contribute to SAMe's efficacy. (1 mg each per day should be sufficient.) As these two vitamins are both safe and part of any healthy diet, it makes perfect sense to make them part of a SAMe program. Also, although it has never been proven that vitamin C and the minerals calcium, magnesium, and potassium help treat the disease, there is no known way that these hinder SAMe's activity and they are, of course, part of any healthy diet.

How strong is the scientific evidence that SAMe works as a treatment for osteoarthritis?

Very, very good—though not conclusive enough for some American researchers and physicians.

First, let us consider animal studies (putting aside all questions of the ethics of using animals in medical experiments). In one study, chickens were injected in both knee joints with a substance causing degeneration of cartilage; then their right knee joints were injected with SAMe (their uninjected left knee joints served as controls). At the end of the test period, the right knees showed significantly less deterioration than the left knees.

A similar experiment using rabbits—animals which are closer to humans in both anatomical and DNA structure—showed even more impressive results. This time, not only was there significantly less deterioration of cartilage tissue in the SAMe-treated joints, but there was also a measurable increase in proteoglycan—physical proof that SAMe promoted the growth of cartilage in the affected areas.

Human studies, of course, cannot provide us with the same kind of objective test results that animal studies can. For example, we cannot inject humans with a specific amount of a substance that causes degeneration of cartilage in order to keep our degeneration rate quantifiable; more significantly, we cannot perform surgery (or post mortems) on human subjects for the sole purpose of measuring deterioration of cartilage tissue or regeneration of proteoglycan. On the other hand, we can do one critical assessment with human subjects that we cannot with animal subjects: We can ask them if they feel better, how much better, and in what specific ways. Furthermore, we can objectively measure some results of therapies with imaging devices such as X rays, CAT scans, and EMIs.

The most extensive human study of SAMe's effects on osteoarthritis depend primarily on subjective, reports of the test subjects, and this is the primary reason that some scientists—mostly American scientists—feel that the results are not sufficiently thorough. But before reviewing this particular study, allow me this comment: If I, personally, suffer from the pain, stiffness, and immobility of osteoarthritis, my main interest is in the subjective results of a treatment—I want to feel and be better, no matter how I come to feel and be that way! Obviously, I can understand the scientists' preoccupation with objective data, the measurements of cartilage tissue deterioration and regrowth. But if as a result of a particular treatment a significant number of people report that they are, for all intents and purposes, cured, this objective data is of only secondary interest to me.

But onto the major human study to date: In a major clinical trial in Germany, 20,621 people suffering from osteoarthritis of the knee, hip, spine, and fingers, were treated for eight weeks with SAMe (600 mg per day for the first two weeks; 400 mg per day for the next two weeks; 200 mg per day for the succeeding four weeks). At the end of this eight-week period, 71% of the subjects self-reported "good" or "very good" results in relieving symptoms of pain, stiffness, and mobility; 21% self-reported "moderate" results of same; and only 9% reported "poor" results (2.3% dropped out due to lack of perceivable benefit). Eighty-seven percent reported perfect tolerance of the drug, while 5% dropped out of the study due to intolerance of the drug (roughly the same percentage that drops out for intolerance in a placebo study).

The sheer number of participants in this study—over 20,000!—makes it a reliable indicator. Also, the protocols (operating standards) of the study were up to snuff by American criteria. What are lacking in the study are control groups and comparative groups (testees taking other drugs, say aspirin or an NSAID). But all that said, the results are impressive to even the most skeptical: More than 70% reported significant alleviation of symptoms of osteoarthritis!

A second impressive study, also at a German university, involved far fewer participants—only 108 subjects—but over a far longer period of time—two years. The subjects suffered from arthritic symptoms in the knee, hip, and spine (not fingers). They began with doses of SAMe of 200 mg three times per day for two weeks, followed thereafter with a maintenance dosage of 200 mg twice per day. Eighty-five percent to 90% of the testees self-reported "good" or "very good" results of the treatment (most reporting significant improvement after only two weeks), and only 5% reported either poor or negative results. Generally, the patients' reports noted a major decrease in morning stiffness and in pain and discomfort both in motion and at rest. Not a single testee dropped out due to unwelcome side effects. And at the end of two years, still no unwelcome side effects appeared. Unsurprisingly, many self-reports spontaneously noted an elevation in mood that the patients attributed to being free from symptoms of their disease. Could this improvement also have been SAMe's antidepressant effect?

Again, this study lacks both controls and comparisons. But nonetheless the protocols were highly respectable and the results supremely impressive for an extended period of time.

Fortunately, some subsequent human studies have had both control and comparison components. Two of these compared treatment with SAMe with treatment with the NSAID naproxen. Again, both studies involved osteoarthritis patients affected at the hip, spine, and knee. The first of these involved 20 subjects over a six-week period; the second, conducted at a major university in Italy, involved 734 people over a 28-day period. The SAMe group took 400 mg three times per day to start, then reduced to 400 mg twice a day. The naproxen group took 250 mg of the NSAID three times a day to start, then reduced to 250 mg twice a day. Finally, to complete double-blind protocols, a third group took a placebo.

Results were consistent in both studies: Patients reported significant improvement of symptoms in roughly equal numbers for SAMe and naproxen. Unsurprisingly, the naproxen subjects reported a significant amount of gastrointestinal disturbance while the SAMe subjects reported virtually none (actually, less than those on the placebo treatment). The doctors authoring the larger study stated that on the basis of the results and SAMe's remarkable tolerableness, they ranked SAMe as a superior treatment for osteo-arthritis.

Similar control and comparative studies were done comparing SAMe with another NSAID, ibuprofen, one with 36 subjects, the other with 150 patients, both over a period of four weeks. The results were virtually identical to the SAMe/naproxen studies. Ditto for two studies comparing SAMe with another NSAID, indomethacin, one involving 36 patients, the other involving 90 patients, both over a period of eight weeks. (Interestingly, the study involving 90 patients included some patients suffering from the other most prevalent form of arthrititis, rheumatoid arthritis; results confirmed that SAMe has *no* effect on that disease.) In another comparison of SAMe treatment with yet another NSAID, piroxicam, the results also showed identical pain-relief and anti-inflammatory action of the two drugs, but with SAMe clearly superior in terms of unwelcome side effects. Two related results from this last experiment are worth noting: While the piroxicam "kicked in" earlier than the SAMe, the effects of SAMe lasted longer after discontinuance than did those of piroxicam after discontinuance. This suggests that SAMe's cartilage-rebuilding component may have contributed to the longer effect.

When it comes to objective data in human studies, the pickings are relatively slim, although there are many such experiments currently in progress, both in Europe and in this country. In one documented double-blind study conducted in Germany using 21 patients suffering from osteoarthritis of the fingers, 14 patients were given 400 mg of SAMe per day while seven received a placebo. At the conclusion of three months, all were given MRIs (Magnetic Resonance Imaging) in the affected areas and those given SAMe showed a significant regrowth of cartilage as compared to those receiving the placebo, who showed no regrowth of cartilage. The number of subjects in this study was too small for drawing any hard and fast conclusions, but combined with the results of the animal studies, the evidence is at the very least strongly suggestive that SAMe promotes cartilage regrowth in people suffering from osteoarthritis.

Considering that some scientists believe that not enough evidence of SAMe's efficacy is in, should I still consider taking SAMe for my osteoarthritis?

Ultimately, this is really only an economic question,

to wit, are you willing to spend the money on SAMe as a treatment even though it has not been proven beyond any doubt to work? Surely, there is sufficient evidence that there are no medical risks involved in taking this substance, so the only risk is economic. (Of course, some physicians will argue that by taking a relatively "untested" drug when you could be taking a tested one, you are putting yourself at an unnecessary risk. However, this argument would only make sense if the "tested" drugs actually worked— and worked without considerable unwelcome side effects!)

At what time of day and how much SAMe should I take to treat osteoarthritis?

SAMe should be taken on an empty stomach, ideally a half hour or more before meals. Also, it is best to take SAMe at regular intervals two or three times a day, rather than all at once.

As to the amount of SAMe that should be taken, doctors' opinions differ, varying from 400 mg per day to 1,600 mg per day. One prominent German physician suggests starting at a relatively high dose of 800 mg per day (400 mg twice a day) for the first two weeks to jumpstart treatment, then reduce to a maintenance dosage of 400 mg per day (200 mg twice a day) thereafter. (For older patients, who may be more sensitive to new medicines, he suggests beginning with the maintenance dosage.)

An American physician, Dr. Michael Murray, recommends starting with a dosage of 400 mg per day (200 mg twice a day) for the first two weeks, upping to 1,200 mg per day (400 mg three times a day) for the next two weeks, and then coming down to maintenance of 400 mg per day again.

Fortunately, you can titrate your personal dosage according to your experience with the drug. If at 400 mg per day you experience full relief from the pain, stiffness, and immobility of osteoarthritis, you will probably choose to stay at that dosage. If you experience only partial relief at that dosage, you will want to raise the dosage until you experience, full relief. Cost will inevitably factor into your choice of dosage. As we will see, SAMe is not cheap. Further, as an over-the-counter drug, it is only rarely covered by medical insurance.

Does this mean that I will have to take SAMe for the rest of my life to enjoy lifelong relief from my osteoarthritis?

Probably. Although because SAMe reverses the progress of osteoarthritis by rebuilding damaged cartilage, you may be able to lower your dosage over the years (no tests have proven this yet, however). You can always "take a vacation" from SAMe usage to see if symptoms return; and if they do, return to it. But for those who find a new lease on life after years of suffering from osteoarthritis, the idea of remaining nonstop on SAMe will probably not feel like such a burden.

How soon will I feel the effects of SAMe?

Most test subjects report relief within two to four weeks.

Is it possible to overdose on SAMe?

No instances of serious effects at high doses have been reported.

Are there any drug interactions with SAMe that I should be aware of?

Only one: the MAO inhibitor antidepressants. (SAMe is just one of a 10-page list of foods and medications that should not be taken with this drug.)

Considering that SAMe appears to stimulate cartilage production, should people without osteoarthritis take it to prevent the onset of this disease?

Common sense would suggest taking SAMe prophylactically (to prevent disease), especially because there are no known unwelcome side effects. But no long-term studies have been conducted that prove SAMe's prophylactic effects with regard to osteoarthritis. And again, the expense is high for this type of use.

PART III

SAMe and Fibromyalgia

ELEVEN

Fibromyalgia: What Is It and Who Gets It?

What is fibromyalgia?

Fibromyalgia is a rather mysterious disease with no definitive origin or cause, nor any conclusive way of diagnosing it. Some medical dictionaries do not even list it. And it has been called by some physicians (rather derisively) "a bunch of symptoms in search of a disease."

Nonetheless, an estimated six to ten million Americans report that they suffer from this particular "bunch" of quite painful and debilitating symptoms, making it the third most frequently seen condition by rheumatologists. Two thirds of sufferers are women; the majority of sufferers are between the ages of 30 and 60, with the median age of those afflicted being 50.

What is this "bunch" of symptoms?

First, there is chronic pain located in fibrous tissue (hence the name). This pain can become so extreme that it becomes difficult for the sufferer to perform any activity. The pain may also come and go for long or short periods with no discernable pattern, at times feeling like the aches of a flu, other times feeling like the extreme tenderness of an injury.

The second most common symptom is arthritis-like stiffness in the muscle tissue, including muscle tissue related to the joints. For this reason, fibromyalgia is sometimes initially diagnosed as some form of arthritis, though subsequent visualization of joint cartilage via X rays or MRIs reveal that it is not.

Next is general fatigue that can become so overwhelming that sufferers often have to give up their work. In this regard, fibromyalgia is similar to the equally mysterious and difficult-to-diagnose disease, chronic fatigue syndrome.

Along with general fatigue, sufferers commonly experience sleep disturbances. Tests have shown that people with fibromyalgia get significantly fewer hours of REM (rapid eye movement) sleep, the level of sleep necessary to allow our nervous systems to be fully alert and in working order the next day. And looking at it from the other direction, if experimental subjects are deprived of REM sleep, after several days they begin to develop fibromyalgia-like symptoms.

Another common symptom of fibromyalgia is depression, and herein lies both some controversy about the disease and some clues as to why SAMe may be the best treatment for it.

The controversy revolves around the old chicken-and-egg argument of "Which came first, the depression or the fibromyalgia?" Because most sufferers of fibromyalgia are middle-aged women who are prone to depression for a variety of reasons, hormonal and otherwise, some doctors (usually male doctors) assume that the symptoms of fatigue, sleep disorder, and general malaise are a *result* of the depression. Others believe that the depression and these other symptoms are all part of a constellation of symptoms of a single-cause disease, while still others believe that the depression is a result of the other debilitating effects of the disease. (In a sense, of course, all three theories could be true.) Clues to why SAMe's antidepressant effect may help relieve many of fibromyalgia's symptoms will be discussed later.

Another mind/mood symptom of fibromyalgia is mental lassitude or fogginess—another symptom that some doctors pin on female middle-aged melancholia. Chronic headaches are often associated with this symptom.

Finally, the extensive list of associated symptoms include chemical sensitivities, morning stiffness (again a symptom that makes it appear like a form of arthritis), numbness and tingling in the extremities, vision disorders, allergies, gastrointestinal disorders (some of which can probably be attributed to the analgesics and NSAIDs that sufferers of fibromyalgia often take to relieve their aches and pains), bladder pain and weakness, and chronic vaginal yeast infections.

How exactly do you diagnose fibromyalgia?

Not easily. And some would say, not at all. At one time, when it was assumed that fibromyalgia was a rheumatological disease that manifests itself in muscle tissue, the patient was tested with electromyography (EMG) and/or tissue biopsies for tissue pathology or inflammation. But these tests consistently showed negative results, adding to some doctors' suspicions that fibromyalgia was "all in the head." Similarly, other visualization techniques such as X rays, EMIs, and CAT scans could not turn up deteriorating or inflamed muscle tissue in the painful areas.

Further, blood and urine tests do not turn up fibromyalgia markers of any kind or any identifiable precursors. In addition, the few (and only occasional) manifest physical symptoms of fibromyalgia—sore throat and swollen lymph nodes—are very common symptoms of any number of transient diseases, including garden-variety flus and allergies.

The reason for this dearth of diagnostic procedures for detecting fibromyalgia is that there is no known cause of fibromyalgia. So what we are left with are only symptoms and patients reporting these symptoms.

It should be noted that in an attempt to come up with a diagnostic procedure with some claim to "objectivity," the American College of Rheumatology has devised something called the "Tender Point Examination," wherein the doctor applies pressure to 18 particular sites on the patient's body—most of them around the neck, knees, elbows, and hips—and the patient reports the degree of pain she experiences from this pressure. If eleven of those 18 points are sensitive and the patient claims that these particular points have been sensitive for at least three months, a diagnosis of fibromyalgia is made.

Obviously, the "Tender Point Examination" is a rather arbitrary diagnostic device (Why 18 points and not ten or nine?) and one that ultimately depends on subjective evaluation at that.

Well, if you cannot diagnose fibromyalgia, how can you call it a disease?

Some doctors would say that exactly for that reason you cannot call fibromyalgia a disease at all. But try telling that to the six to ten million Americans who suffer from that "bunch of symptoms in search of a disease." Their chronic and often extreme pain is real to them, whether or not science can pinpoint its cause or visualize its "damage" to the body. Ditto for the chronic fatigue and sleeping disorders, the stiffness, depression, and all of the other attendant "subjective" symptoms that these millions suffer from. Like chronic fatigue syndrome and Gulf War syndrome (two diseases that some doctors believe are organically related to fibromyalgia), fibromyalgia basically can only be defined by its symptoms. But because the sheer number of people suffering from these symptoms is so large and their symptoms so consistent among this large group, it would not only be medically obtuse to deny that it is a disease, it would be morally irresponsible to do so.

Still, there is one other way we can define and diagnose fibromyalgia—by what alleviates its symptoms. We will discuss these treatments in the next two chapters, but first a few words about the practice of defining a disease by its cures.

Many purists believe that this is a backward approach to medical diagnosis, one that risks "creating" new diseases out of a drug's effects. For example, once it was found that the stimulant Ritalin aided problem students in attending to their schoolwork, a new definition of the mental disorder/disease Attention Deficit Disorder (ADD) was born—children who "responded well" to Ritalin suffered from ADD. In this way, the population of children suffering from this "disease" expanded tenfold and many people believe that this is a dangerous trend. However, in the case of fibromyalgia, with its undeniable and debilitating physical component, any drug that reduces or eradicates the symptoms is worth our consideration whether or not it is used to "define" the disease.

Are there any current theories about what causes fibromyalgia?

Yes, and some of them are quite interesting. Many scientists hypothesize that fibromyalgia is what is called a *systemic* disorder involving both the central nervous system (CNS) and the endocrine (hormonal) system—systems that are, of course, closely connected to one another. One of the places where these two systems intersect is the limbic system (neurons involved in the sleep-wake cycle), which is directed by the hypothalamus gland; many doctors believe that fibromyalgia is a disorder of the limbic system. Still other scientists add the immune system to this list of possible systemic disorders responsible for this mysterious ailment.

What most of these theories have in common is that they postulate disruption in the brain's capacity for regulating the following crucial body functions: the sleep-wake cycle, body temperature (disorders of which can result in tissue pain), hormone production, flow of blood to the brain (obstruction of which can result in disturbances in pain perception), and the autonomic (involuntary) nervous system. Each one of these offers suggestions for treatment of fibromyalgia.

TWELVE

The Most Common Treatments
for Fibromyalgia

*What treatments do doctors most commonly prescribe
for fibromyalgia?*

Doctors usually prescribe painkillers, anti-inflammatories, muscle relaxants, sleep aids and sleep stabi-
lizers, exercise, stress reduction, and psychological
treatments.

For obvious reasons, each of these treatments
addresses individual symptoms and symptoms only,
and for that reason various combinations of these
treatments are often prescribed for a patient.

*What are the most commonly prescribed painkillers,
anti-inflammatories, and muscle relaxants?*

The usual suspects when it comes to painkillers and
anti-inflammatories: aspirin and other analgesics, the
various NSAIDs, and sometimes steroids. As we have

seen in our discussion of osteoarthritis, every one of these options is a mixed blessing at best. Yes, pain is often significantly reduced, but in the case of aspirin and other analgesics (e.g., acetaminophen) and the NSAIDs, common unwelcome side effects include serious gastrointestinal disorders (often leading to ulcers), internal bleeding (including bleeding ulcers), and the possibility of kidney and liver damage. Likewise, steroids may significantly reduce the pain of fibromyalgia, but at the risk of serious hormonal disorders.

Some synthetic opiates, like Ultram, have proved effective pain relievers and soporifics (sleeping aids) for people suffering from fibromyalgia. Again, the price one pays for continued use of opiates includes clouded thinking and the possibility of addiction.

Muscle relaxants have shown themselves to be a boon for many sufferers of fibromyalgia. Among those most frequently prescribed are Flexeril and Robaxin; the over-the-counter muscle relaxant Aleve has also shown promise for people with mild cases of fibromyalgia. The side effects of this class of drugs are still being catalogued, but many steady users complain of chronic weakness and fatigue—two of the most common symptoms of the disease itself!

What are the most commonly prescribed sleeping aids for fibromyalgia?

Again, it is the usual suspects, and therein lies a considerable danger. Some doctors prescribe the popular sleeping pill Halcion to fibromyalgia patients who complain of night after night of inadequate sleep followed by increased pain and stiffness. But there are many known problems with this medication, the most alarming of which is that it induces depression in a significant number of users. Here, again, we have a case of a drug relieving one symptom of the disease while exacerbating another symptom of that disease! Further, some researchers now believe that Halcion does not provide truly restful and restorative (REM) sleep, so it does not even fully address the problems related to sleeplessness. (It may well be that Halcion's proclivity for inducing depression is related to the fact that it bypasses REM sleep.)

Over-the-counter and alternative sleeping aids such as valerian root, kava-kava, and 5-HTP are also used by sufferers from fibromyalgia with varying results. Again, many patients complain that while they sleep better and enjoy lower levels of stress when taking these preparations, their energy levels during waking hours is not improved at all—in fact, some believe it reduces their energy levels. Finally, some people suffering from fibromyalgia have begun experimenting with the over-the-counter hormone supplement, melatonin, which addresses sleeping problems by working directly on the sleep-wake cycle. Melatonin also has been known to improve mild depression. So far, the jury is out on the use of melatonin in this regard.

Is exercise really helpful for people with fibromyalgia?

You bet, as important as it is for people suffering from arthritis. And as with that disease, the temptation to slip into a life of total inactivity to avoid pain only leads to increased pain and stiffness. Again, as with arthritis, an exercise program that combines stretching with aerobics not only makes the affected muscles more pliable and stronger, it targets the muscle group for more oxygenation and cellular regeneration.

For a total muscle workout with low impact, swimming regularly is by far the best option. And for low-stress stretching, yoga is the exercise of choice for most people who suffer from fibromyalgia. (Yoga and meditation can also help one improve his tolerance for pain which, from a subjective point of view, is about the same as pain reduction.)

Again, as with arthritis, massage of various types—especially shiatsu and acupressure massage—can help keep muscles loose and pliable while reducing pain, especially if massage is done in conjunction with an exercise regime. And finally, postural adjustments like chiropractics and postural exercises like the Alexander Method have been known to help in controlling the symptoms of this disease.

How does stress reduction affect fibromyalgia?

Stress reduction goes a long way in reducing the symptoms of this disease, just as we are now discovering that stress reduction goes a long way in reducing the symptoms of a whole host of diseases. Basically, stress reduction has the indirect effect of boosting up the immune system, thus reducing deterioration of all vital cells, tissues, and organs. So whatever it is that has gone amiss in sufferers of fibromyalgia, a hearty immune system helps to counter its adverse effects.

But we must add to this the fact that in a statistically significant number of individuals, onset of fibromyalgia has followed directly from periods of intense stress. Ditto for increased pain and symptoms of this disease. This fact certainly suggests that at the very least a highly stressed individual is more susceptible to the disease than others, possibly because her immune system is in poorer shape. So the advisability of a stress-reduction program for fibromyalgia sufferers is obvious.

Yoga, as we have said, goes a long way in helping us to reduce stress, as do active exercise and massage. But stress reduction really has to be a way of life to be effective. By this I mean that we have to learn how to stop our daily anxieties and worries and compulsions in their tracks. We need to restructure our thinking and feeling in our daily lives to be more "easy does it" and less "got to do it." Easier said than done, of course. But yoga, exercise, and massage help you set up this new mindset. So can meditation exercises like those suggested by Transcendental Meditation, which offer you a "tranquil mind" for set periods each day. And then, of course, there are antianxiety prescription drugs and over-the-counter preparations like kava-kava and St. John's wort, although as I have noted, both of these types of drugs may also contribute to the lethargy that is one of the symptoms of the disease. Finally, of course, there is psychological therapy of various kinds, which we consider below.

Is depression the cause of fibromyalgia or is it an effect of the disease?

Possibly both. Depression and stressed-out feelings, of course, are two sides of the same coin, so a depressed person is probably more likely to be susceptible to fibromyalgia than other people, just as a highly stressed person is more susceptible to the disease than others. But also there is no doubt that fibromyalgia is a "depressing" disease—to suffer day in and out from an ailment that leaves you in pain, immobile, and without energy is bound to do considerable damage to your zest for life. So it is likely that when it comes to depression and fibromyalgia, we are confronted with a vicious cycle: Depression begets fibromyalgia, which begets depression, which exacerbates the symptoms of fibromyalgia . . . and on and on.

Still, it would be a mistake to say that depression is the sole cause of fibromyalgia. Statistical evidence simply does not bear this out in any meaningful way. Why, for example, does only some small percentage of those suffering from depression also have the symptoms associated with fibromyalgia? No one has answered this rather basic question satisfactorily to date.

On the other hand, the association between the two conditions is usually strong. Sleep disturbances, headaches, and general fatigue are symptoms common to both diseases. Sufferers from fibromyalgia have disproportionate family histories of depression. And most importantly, fibromyalgia patients have found significant—though only transient—relief from most symptoms of the disease by taking small doses of prescription antidepressants, particularly the tricyclics Elavil (amitriptyline), Norpamin (desipramine), and Anafranil (clomipramine). Unfortunately, the operative word here is *transient*—in the great majority of cases the anti-depressants lose their effectiveness within months.

A danger in equating depression with fibromyalgia is that it adds to the "it's all in your head" thinking that dogs this undiagnosable disease. This kind of thinking appears to particularly attach itself to diseases that attack more women than men, part of the "women are victims of their own emotions" bias prevalent in the male-dominated medical and medical research profession. The outcome of this kind of thinking is to not take patients' complaints seriously.

Still, does psychological therapy help control fibromyalgia?

It can. An effective course of psychotherapy often reduces stress and, as we have seen, stress can make a person susceptible to this disease. Furthermore, in as much as depression is itself a symptom of fibromyalgia, psychotherapy can go a long way in reducing this particular symptom. This can reverse the vicious depression-fibromyalgia-depression cycle in telling ways. For example, a fibromyalgia patient who is depressed is less likely to embark on an ameliorative exercise program than an undepressed patient is.

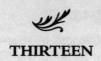

THIRTEEN

The SAMe Treatment
for Fibromyalgia

How does SAMe treat fibromyalgia?

In a remarkable number of cases, SAMe addresses two major symptoms of fibromyalgia: depression and muscle soreness. And it has proved effective in these two areas without the unwelcome side effects associated with prescription antidepressants (see Chapter 5) or the unwelcome side effects of analgesics and anti-inflammatories (see Chapter 9). Further, some test studies show that SAMe also relieves the common fibromyalgia symptoms of morning stiffness, fatigue, and sleep disorders.

However—and for some sufferers from fibromyalgia, this is a very big "however"—treatment with SAMe does not appear to relieve sensitivity at tender points or muscle weakness.

Furthermore, a meta-analysis of test studies done on SAMe and fibromyalgia show inconsistent results on SAMe's effectiveness in relieving fibromyalgia-related depression. In other words, just like the disease itself, the effectiveness of this promising treatment remains at least partly unclear.

How does SAMe relieve the muscle soreness of fibromyalgia?

Apparently in pretty much the same way as it relieves the soreness of osteoarthritis: by serving as both a painkiller and anti-inflammatory.

As you may recall, SAMe is intimately involved with transsulfuration, a process that produces a supremely important substance in our bodies called glutathione. And glutathione is a proven natural anti-inflammatory in our bodies.

It is worth noting here that some doctors hypothesize that SAMe actually offers a protective effect against the progression of fibromyalgia due to the "master antioxidant" properties of glutathione: by reducing the number of free radicals circulating in the body, glutathione makes the immune system more powerful and, as fibromyalgia seems to prey on weakened immune systems, glutathione therefore protects against this disease.

How does SAMe counter depression in fibromylagia patients (that is, when it works)?

Apparently in the same way it counters depression in other depressives: by boosting the brain population of the critical neurotransmitters melatonin, serotonin, and dopamine.

As you may recall, SAMe achieves this by promoting methylation on three different fronts: by regulating the breakdown of the neurotransmitters (protein methylation), by speeding production of the receptor molecules the neurotransmitters attach themselves to (DNA methylation), and by making existing receptor molecules more responsive (phospholipid methylation).

The last of these methylation processes, phospholipid methylation, is probably the most significant. When the membranes of nerve cells are incapable of accepting such neurotransmitters as serotonin or dopamine, depression is sure to follow. But SAMe-induced phospholipid methylation stimulates the production of phospholipids which, in turn, keep nerve membranes in tiptop condition, making them more able to accept these critical, mood-affecting neurotransmitters.

Another way in which SAMe controls depression in fibromylagia patients is by regulating stress hormones such as adrenaline. In this way, SAMe packs a double whammy of reducing depression and reducing anxiety, which is a direct link to the stress that seems to be at least one of the precipitating conditions, if not its cause of fibromylagia.

Finally, we should note that SAMe's antidepressant effects on fibromylagia patients appear to last for a longer period than those of the common prescription antidepressants (and, of course, without their side effects). But again, the test evidence here remains too scant to be conclusive.

Okay, what is the scientific evidence for SAMe's efficacy as a treatment for fibromylagia?

To date, there are four major studies of the effects of SAMe on all symptoms of fibromylagia. None of these studies were done with significantly large populations of subjects.

A double-blind study done in Denmark involved 44 fibromyalgia patients, half of whom were given placebos and half 800 mg per day of SAMe. The study lasted six weeks, and at the end of that period the SAMe group showed significantly more improvement in terms of pain, fatigue, and morning stiffness. The SAMe group also showed improvement in sleep patterns, possibly as a result of the pain reduction. However, there was no significant improvement in sensitivity at tender points, muscle strength or elasticity, or depression as measured by a self-reporting test (Beck Depression Inventory). As always, the SAMe group experienced no side effects of any kind.

A double-blind study done in Italy involved only 17 fibromyalgia patients, 11 of whom suffered from accompanying depression. In the first phase, part of the group was administered 200 mg per day of SAMe for 21 days while a control group was given a placebo for the same period, then results were calculated for both groups; in the second phase (after a "rest" period of two weeks), the two groups and dosages were switched. Both phases showed significant relief for the SAMe group in terms of pain in trigger points and in depressions. But I repeat, the number of participants in this study is woefully small.

Another double-blind Scandinavian study involved 34 fibromylagia patients, half of whom received 600 mg per day of SAMe and half a placebo. The results of this study were less impressive: a significant, but relatively small improvement in SAMe group in pain both at rest and in movement, and in fatigue, sleep, and mood, but no difference at all in tender point sensitivity or muscle strength and pliability.

Finally, there is another Italian study, this one involving 47 fibromylagia patients. The results showed marked improvement in the SAMe-taking group of testees in the areas of pain, sleep disorders, and mood, but none in tender point sensitivity or muscle strength and pliability.

Is the evidence strong enough to take SAMe for fibromylagia?

This is a personal judgment call. On the one hand, the overall test evidence is relatively scant. But on the other hand, SAMe has no known unwelcome side effects, so the risk you take is strictly economic (that is, if you do not count the risk of failed hopes).

If your most pronounced symptoms of fibromylagia are depression, pain, and sleep disruption—or if treating these symptoms out of many is significant for you—you will probably want to take this economic risk.

Can you take SAMe with other fibromyalgia medications or treatments?

Again, with the exception of MAO inhibitors (a low-choice antidepressant), the answer is yes.

At what time of day and how much SAMe should I take for fibromyalgia?

Most doctors recommend the same dosage regime as for depression patients: Start with a daily dosage of 400 mg (two doses of 200 mg). Take the supplement on an empty stomach at least one half hour before a meal. Because SAMe-induced methylation will not work with low levels of vitamin B_{12} or folic acid, a 1 mg supplement of each of these is recommended in conjunction with SAMe.

If after 21 days, you do not feel that your symptoms have been sufficiently reduced, add another 400 mg daily dose of SAMe to be taken on an empty stomach at a different time of day, for a total of 800 mg per day (four doses of 200 mg). If after another 14 days, you do not feel that your symptoms have been sufficiently reduced, add another 400 mg daily dose as above for a total of 1,200 mg per day (three doses of 400 mg). And if after another 14 days, you still do not feel that your symptoms have been sufficiently reduced, add yet another 400 mg daily dose for a total of 1,600 mg per day (four doses of 400 mg). After another two weeks, if you still do not feel significant relief, SAMe is not the treatment for you.

PART IV

SAMe and Liver Diseases

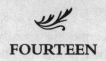

FOURTEEN

What Is Liver Disease and Who Gets It?

What is liver disease?

The most common diseases of the liver are cirrhosis and hepatitis, both of them fairly prevalent in our society and both of them potentially life threatening, although most forms of hepatitis are far less dangerous than cirrhosis. But in order to understand these diseases, we must first understand the nature and function of the liver itself.

THE LIVER

The liver is an essential, multifunctional gland located in the upper-right quadrant of the abdomen. Its primary functions are involved with digestion and the development of erythrocytes, red blood cells responsible for the transportation of oxygen and carbon dioxide. It is critical in detoxifying harmful substances in the blood, producing bile, which metabolizes fats in our digestion, and in storing food in the form of glycogen (a carbohydrate) and fats. In addition, the liver builds many essential blood proteins and stores up some vitamins until they are needed by other organs. The gland is also critical for the production of prothrombin, a substance necessary for clotting blood. Further, the liver is vital in maintaining sex hormones and other steroidal hormone balances in the body.

Unlike any other gland or organ, the liver has the remarkable capacity for regenerating itself. If up to 80% of the liver is damaged or removed (as in a partial-liver transplant), as long as the basic structure of the remaining portion stays intact this organ will regrow to its original size and shape and return to operating at full capacity in a matter of only months. According to some anatomists, this unique capacity of the liver is a primary survival characteristic of the human species. If the liver could not continuously regenerate, it would quickly waste away from all the damage it constantly endures, and humans would have a radically reduced life span.

But despite this miraculous characteristic, the liver is not impervious to lasting damage and destruction, especially to the damage done to it in its function as a detoxifier. And the reason that the liver succumbs to damage done to it while performing this function is that this damage compromises the basic structure of the gland.

So let's take a closer look at the liver's function as a detoxifier. The liver disposes of worn-out blood cells by breaking them down into their different elements, storing the elements that the body will use later and shuttling the rest to the kidneys for disposal in the urine. It filters and destroys bacteria, neutralizes poisons, and rejects and disposes of toxic amino acids generated from protein metabolism.

The most destructive toxins that the liver has to deal with come from airborne toxins in our increasingly poisoned environment and from the foods we eat and drinks we drink. Highest on the list of the latter are the poisons contained in alcohol, especially when consumed in excessive amounts.

Okay, what is cirrhosis of the liver?

Cirrhosis of the liver is chronic scarring of the liver tissue that eventually leads to liver failure and death. The liver cells degenerate and the surrounding tissue thickens, gradually weakening the gland's ability to neutralize and/or dispose of toxins in the body, including those very toxins that are killing liver cells. The body, then, succumbs to these unneutralized, circulating poisons that it cannot dispose of. The nature of the damage done to the liver cells is such that basic structure of the gland is irrevocably changed, thus making regeneration of liver cells impossible.

Men are more likely than women to come down with cirrhosis (by a ratio of 2:1), and the disease usually strikes people of both sexes in their forties and fifties. The most likely candidates for this disease are excessive drinkers; they account for 75% of cirrhosis patients in the United States. The other 25% come down with the disease as a result of damage from hepatitis (B or C), bile duct blockage that causes bile backup (usually as a result of duct scarring or gallstones), chronic pancreatitis (also often a result of excessive alcohol intake), heart disease, or toxic chemicals or drugs (including excessive intake of fat-soluble vitamin supplements, particularly A, D, and E). Some people are genetically predisposed to coming down with cirrhosis, especially those with inherited metabolic disorders that cause toxic buildup of iron and copper in the liver and other organs.

What are the symptoms of cirrhosis?

The initial symptoms are subtle: loss of appetite, fatigue, weakness, and weight loss—in fact, identical to early symptoms of both depression and fibromyalgia. Later comes nausea, vomiting, and abdominal discomfort. Then come changes in the appearance of the skin and eyes including pallor (a sign of anemia), the appearance of small red spots called spider angiomas, reddened palms, dilated capillaries (yes, the kind seen on the faces of alcoholics), and finally jaundice, a yellowing of the skin and eyes as a result of bile buildup.

Along the way, as toxins accumulate, the patient's ability to fight off infections decreases drastically, often resulting in secondary diseases that further deteriorate the body. As a result of the liver's inability to produce adequate amounts of prothrombin (the blood clotter), both internal and external bleeding occurs—frequent and severe nosebleeds, blood in stool, easy bruising (blood under the skin), and bleeding gums. As the scar tissue builds up, the liver may become enlarged and/or tender. As sex hormone production also decreases with impaired liver function, disappearance of menstruation in women, impotence in men, and sterility in both are common symptoms in later stages of the disease. There may be chronic fever in these latter stages as the result of infections that the body can no longer fight. And finally there is progressive sleepiness that ultimately ends with coma and death.

How does alcohol cause this irreparable damage to the liver?

Alcohol does its damage on the liver in a chain reaction that starts at the cellular level, where it compromises mitochondria function and where it is converted into a toxic substance known as acetaldehyde.

As a result of these two cellular events, liver cells build up excessive amounts of fats in the form of fatty acids, which in turn leads directly to the damage that results in scarring and all of the impaired liver function that follows from that scarring.

First, let's take a brief look at the compromised mitochondria function. Mitochondria are an essential part of all living cells that convert glucose into energy. Alcohol poisons the mitochondrion membrane, reducing its ability to accept glucose and thus impairing this entire basic metabolic process.

Next, let's look at how alcohol (ethanol) is converted into acetaldehyde, a dangerous toxin. This is actually only an intermediary step in the detoxification of ethanol; in the final step, ethanol is turned into a harmless and easily disposable form of vinegar. But when this detoxification process is overloaded with ethanol from excessive alcoholic intake, the acetaldehyde does not go to this final step quickly enough. The result is that it lingers in the liver long enough to wreak some real damage. The lingering acetaldehyde reduces the liver's capacity for converting fat into energy; it reduces the kidney's capacity for excreting uric acid (which, in itself, can lead to some forms of arthritis), and it reduces the capacity of the liver to convert glycogen into glucose.

It is in this last disruption where alcohol packs a double whammy to the liver. Not only does it reduce the liver's capacity to produce that basic unit of energy, glucose, but by poisoning the mitochondrial membrane, alcohol decreases the cells' ability to accept what little glucose is produced. This is exactly what leads to the next step in the chain reaction: With little or no conversion of glycogen into glucose taking place in the liver cells, the cells become overloaded with glycogen and accompanying fatty acids. This literally causes cellular fatty buildup, which causes the cells to break down and stop functioning. And this, in turn, results in a situation where the liver cannot deal with *any* of the toxins that it would normally filter or dispose of.

The last step in this downward spiral is the scarring of the liver tissue, the natural result of any cellular breakdown. As the scarring progresses, it starts to block the vital channels in the liver: the bile ducts and its blood vessels. In both cases, backup of the fluids occurs. Bile clogs the liver; and blood not only clogs the liver, impeding all bloodflow through this organ, but it backs up in the spleen, intestines, and extremities where the pressure may become so great that bleeding occurs, including potentially fatal internal bleeding.

The cycle goes on, of course: Excessive bleeding is compounded by the reduced ability to clot blood; bile buildup leads to further impairment of liver function; and unmediated toxin buildup leads to further impairment of liver function, not to mention other organs and glands.

And throughout this process, the liver's vaunted ability to regenerate itself is lost.

What is hepatitis?

Hepatitis is an inflammation of the liver, usually as a secondary symptom of other diseases including amebic dysentery, mononucleosis, and cirrhosis. Unlike cirrhosis, up to 85% of hepatitis patients usually recover with bed rest and diet adjustments. A common form, infectious hepatitis, is a viral infection, often transmitted by contaminated foods and toxins in the environment (for example the waste product, carbon tetrachloride), or more commonly, by contaminated blood and secretions. Another form, serum hepatitis (hepatitis B), also viral, is most often the result of unsterile blood and/or hypodermic needles, hence a prevalent disease among intravenous heroine users. Alcoholic hepatitis is inflammation of the liver due to alcohol poisoning; in this common form, the liver completely loses its ability to neutralize toxins and becomes toxic itself. It is important to note that not only can hepatitis result from cirrhosis, it can also lead to this disease.

What are the symptoms of hepatitis?

The symptoms are similar to those of cirrhosis: loss of appetite, nausea, fatigue, muscle weakness, fever, tenderness and/or enlargement of the liver, and jaundice. Other symptoms may include breast enlargement in men, hair loss, enlarged spleen, fluid accumulation in legs and abdomen, and hallucinations. Severe cases can involve the brain, causing rapid-onset dementia.

A series of blood tests can diagnose hepatitis.

FIFTEEN

The Most Common Treatments for Cirrhosis and Hepatitis

What treatments do doctors most commonly prescribe for cirrhosis?

Unfortunately, this will be a rather short chapter because there is very little in the way of medical treatment that can be offered to patients with this debilitating liver disease.

Treatment of cirrhosis basically consists of avoiding toxic substances, especially those that may have contributed to the onset of the disease (most notably, alcohol consumption), bed rest, a diet that emphasizes proteins, and a diet or supplements that include folic acid, thiamine, pyridoxine, vitamin K, magnesium, and phosphates.

Not all doctors prescribe a high-protein diet. On the one hand, the body of a cirrhosis patient is running on a short supply of blood proteins because the liver has ceased metabolizing them, plus the fact that protein is needed to regenerate liver cells; on the other hand, a buildup of the extremely dangerous poison, ammonia, occurs as a result of the liver's inability to make urea. (This where the hallucinations in hepatitis come from—brain poisoning by ammonia.) Those doctors (the majority) who opt for a high-protein diet recommend 1 g of protein per kilogram of body weight, or approximately 75 to 100 grams of protein per day. The high or low protein conundrum is just one of the lose/lose situations a physician treating liver diseases is confronted with.

The vitamin supplements are especially recommended to patients who have come down with liver disease as a result of excessive alcohol—alcoholics tend to have limited diets (often limited to the drinks themselves) and hence need the vitamin basics. Also, a common complication of cirrhosis is the failure of the liver to make vitamins available in an active form in the body, so for this reason the need for the basic nutrients is also high. Among common vitamin deficiencies in liver disease patients are the fat soluble ones, especially A, but also D and E. But, as we have seen, excessive amounts of these very vitamins can exacerbate the disease—another lose/lose area. Treatment with Vitamin K is an attempt (usually fruitless) to boost the body's failing ability to clot blood and thus to stem internal bleeding associated with these diseases.

Because of the fluid accumulation in the abdomen

and extremities, patients are sometimes given diuretics to increase fluid disposal. (Also for this reason, patients are usually put on a low-sodium diet to avoid further fluid retention.) And because of the risk of ammonia poisoning patients may be given antibiotics to stem ammonia build-up. Both of these treatments, of course, are only addressing symptoms and secondary problems of the diseases, not the diseases themselves.

The current treatment of last resort for cirrhosis is a liver transplant, a surgical procedure that is fraught with all the complications and risks of any transplant surgery, beginning with the problem of finding a suitable donor. However, because of the liver's remarkable ability to regenerate from as little of 20% of its original mass, *partial liver transplants from living donors* are becoming the most promising procedure for replacing a hopelessly damaged liver. This new procedure involves removing a section of the liver from a DNA-compatible donor and transplanting it to the site of the liver of the diseased patient. There it is provided with an environment that promotes regrowth, which is exactly what it does: A healthy liver regrows in place of the diseased and deteriorating one.

What treatments do doctors most commonly prescribe for hepatitis?

Again, avoiding the offending toxin or toxins, bed rest, and vitamin supplements head the list. Some doctors prescribe Interferon for hepatitis C with varying degrees of success, but at the risk of causing severe Interferon-induced depression. Some alternative physicians believe that megadoses of vitamin C cut the recovery time from this disease in half.

A vaccine for serum hepatitis (hepatitis B) is highly recommended for people who will be travelling in Third World countries and people who have sexual contact with people suffering from this disease.

SIXTEEN

The SAMe Treatment for Cirrhosis and Hepatitis

How does SAMe treat cirrhosis?

Very well indeed! Treatment with SAMe appears to actually reverse the damage done to the liver by cirrhosis. And it does this with a four-pronged attack: It improves the liver's capacity for metabolizing substances; it improves the liver's capacity for generating proteins; it improves the capacity of the mitochondria in the liver's cells to accept substances; and ultimately, it stimulates the liver to regenerate itself!

Let's start by looking at the fundamental relationship between SAMe and the liver. More than half of the eight grams of SAMe that a normal body produces each day is synthesized in the liver. That is because the liver is highly dependent on SAMe to perform many of its basic functions, including regeneration of its own tissue.

Looking at this from the opposite direction, patients suffering from cirrhosis almost invariably display very low SAMe levels. To understand why this happens, recall that the body manufactures its own SAMe by combining the amino acid methionine with the energy molecule ATP. Key to this combining process is the naturally produced enzyme, S-adenosylmethionine synthetase (literally, the SAMe synthesizing enzyme). But one substantial piece of damage done by cirrhosis is to curtail production of SAMe synthetase. As a result, the methionine remains unattached to the ATP and starts to build up in the system, becoming a powerful toxin itself. A second and very harmful result is that without the synthesized SAMe, the liver cannot produce the bile that metabolizes fats with the result of fatty buildup in the liver and all the serious damage that follows from that. Further and perhaps most importantly, without SAMe the liver is unable to produce the antioxidant glutathione, causing the free radicals to multiply and abet the proliferation of toxins in the body, including in the liver itself.

The various methylation processes that are dependent on SAMe also have a direct connection to liver function. As you may remember, *protein methylation* is necessary for cellular health—both cell growth and cell repair—and that includes the cells of the liver. Furthermore, both *protein and phospholipid methylation* activate cell membrane receptors. In alcohol-related cirrhosis, alcohol poisons the mitochondrion membrane in the liver cells, reducing its ability to accept glucose and thus impairing this entire basic metabolic process. But SAMe, if it is in the system, can refurbish and reactivate these membranes, allowing them to accept glucose and get the metabolic process back on track. And finally, DNA methylation is necessary for activating genes which, in turn, are necessary for regulating cell growth, repair, and reproduction. DNA methylation regulates these processes in the liver, just as it does in other parts of the body. Without adequate DNA methylation, liver cells are "poorly managed," resulting in inefficient cell repair and sluggish cell reproduction.

Put all of this together and it is evident that if you add SAMe to your system in order to make up for SAMe decline as a result of cirrhosis damage, you end up reversing much of cirrhosis's damage to your liver and body.

Are you saying that SAMe supplements address the symptoms of cirrhosis or that they address the disease itself?

In a sense, both. Treatment with SAMe supplements restarts critical processes that have been stopped by the cirrhosis. But these processes—the production of bile to dissolve fats, the disposal of various toxins, including methionine and others that damage the liver itself, and the various methylations that maintain and regenerate liver cells—are not only necessary for general health, they are necessary for the health of the liver itself. As cirrhosis is a chain-reaction of damaging effects, the introduction of SAMe short-circuits this chain reaction, permitting the liver to heal and regenerate rather than succumb to the effects of its own disease.

How does treatment with SAMe compare with conventional treatments for cirrhosis?

Very well, but let's face it, there isn't any competition to speak of. Certainly, it is the *only* treatment for cirrhosis that can claim to actually reverse the damage done to the liver by this disease.

Should SAMe treatment for cirrhosis be done in conjunction with any other therapies?

Yes. For starters, it makes no sense to embark on any treatment for cirrhosis while continuing to drink alcohol or to expose yourself to any other toxins that may be the original cause of the disease. The good news here for habitual or addictive drinkers is that SAMe, like other medicines with an antidepressant effect, makes it much easier to ease yourself away from alcohol dependancy. With depression under control, you will no longer have the need to "blot out the (emotional) pain" with alcohol.

Bed rest is important for recovery from any serious disease and cirrhosis is no exception. It allows the body to "concentrate" its energy on healing. The various regenerative effects of SAMe will be given a far better chance of working if your energy is not being expended in any other way.

A diet that emphasizes proteins can help here also, as protein is needed to regenerate liver cells once the SAMe gets this process going again. And taking SAMe significantly reduces the risk of toxic ammonia buildup due to unmetabolized protein because the SAMe also gets that process back on track again.

Finally, a diet or supplements that include folic acid, thiamine, pyridoxine, vitamin K, magnesium, and phosphates can possibly help in the overall healing process, while the folic acid and B_{12} help revitalize internal SAMe production. In reasonable amounts, certainly none of these supplements can do any harm.

How strong is the scientific evidence that SAMe works as a treatment for cirrhosis?

Very, very good—although long-term studies are yet to be conducted. But short-term studies offer strong objective evidence that SAMe supplements address several critical aspects of this disease.

Restores bile function. Several studies have demonstrated that adding SAMe supplements to the diet of cirrhosis patients significantly increased production of the taurine element (another product of SAMe transsulfuration) of bile salts with the end result of restoring bile function. This, of course, meant that fats could once again be metabolized by the liver, putting an end to the deadly fatty buildup in that organ. One such study, reported in the *Scandinavian Journal of Clinical and Laboratory Investigation*, showed that a dosage of 800 mg per day of SAMe for only two months was enough to significantly increase bile output and outflow.

Boosts glutathione production. Several studies (including the one above) demonstrated that adding SAMe supplements to the diet of cirrhosis patients significantly boosted production of glutathione, the "master antioxidant," thus measurably reducing the amount of toxins circulating in the body and particularly in the liver. These studies showed that every step in this reverse chain reaction worked: but when glutathione was boosted, the population of free radicals declined, as did the population of toxins, with the end result of reduced toxicity in the liver.

Improves liver function. Several double-blind studies in Italy (the country that is clearly in the forefront in applications of SAMe to a variety of ailments) demonstrated that adding SAMe supplements along with vitamin B_{12} to the diet of cirrhosis patients significantly improved measurable liver functions, including protein synthesis (especially albumin), the ability to break down red blood cell products, and the ability to diffuse immune molecules. In one group of studies, patients were given only 180 mg of SAMe per day (30 mg six times per day) along with vitamin

B_{12}; at the end of 30 days, improvement in these three functions was already detectable. In another study, patients were given 150 mg of SAMe daily along with vitamin B_{12}; at the end of only 20 days, protein production of the liver had returned to normal levels.

Increases the ability of mitochondria to accept substances. In a study reported in the journal *Hematology*, researchers demonstrated that adding SAMe to the diet of patients suffering from alcohol-induced cirrhosis improved flow through cellular membranes, including the flow of glutathione into the mitochondria. This means the restoration of a fundamental liver function: the metabolization of glucose.

Improves production and function of red blood cells. In another study of patients suffering from alcohol-induced cirrhosis who were given 2 grams of SAMe per day, a measurable increase in two key components of red blood cell production and function, cysteine and glutathione, were detected.

Putting all of these individual improvements together, we see that adding SAMe to the diet of cirrhosis patients not only restores several critical functions of the liver, but it provides essential elements for regenerating damaged liver cells.

But impressive as the results of these short-term experiments are, we still do not have results of long-term studies that could show full or near full recovery from cirrhosis from SAMe treatment. Undoubtedly, the next several years will bring us those results.

Considering that these long-term studies have not been done yet, should I still consider taking SAMe for cirrhosis?

Again, this is basically only an economic question because there are no medical risks involved in taking SAMe.

At what time of day and how much SAMe should I take to treat cirrhosis?

Ideally, SAMe should be taken under a physician's supervision for this disease, as there are so many variables to consider, such as, whether the disease is alcohol induced, in which higher dosages are usually recommended. Note also that some physicians believe that intravenous administration of both the drug and vitamin B_{12} produces better and faster results.

If taken orally, the usual advice prevails: SAMe should be taken on an empty stomach, ideally a half-hour or more before meals. Also, it is best to take SAMe at regular intervals two or three times a day, rather than all at once.

Most doctors who prescribe SAMe for cirrhosis recommend starting with a relatively high dose, say 800 mg per day, for the first two weeks to jump-start treatment, then reduce to a maintenance dosage of 400 mg per day thereafter and see how things go. But again, when it comes to cirrhosis, a physician's supervision and monitoring of results is the best route to take.

Does this mean that I will have to take SAMe for the rest of my life to enjoy lifelong relief from my cirrhosis?

Possibly not. But again, as SAMe treatment may never fully "cure" the disease but only make it infinitely more manageable, most physicians suggest staying on some maintenance dose of SAMe even after this improvement is seen.

How soon will I experience improvement with SAMe?

Most test subjects report relief within two to four weeks.

How does SAMe treat hepatitis?

In general, SAMe's effects on hepatitis patients are similar to its effects on cirrhosis patients (of course, the two diseases often coexist, one leading to the other).

Few studies have been done on patients suffering only from hepatitis. But promising results have been seen in patients with chronic and/or alcohol-induced hepatitis.

PART V

SAMe and Parkinson's Disease

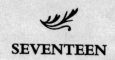

SEVENTEEN

What Is Parkinson's Disease and Who Gets It?

What is Parkinson's disease?

Parkinson's disease is a progressive degenerative disease of the brain, usually occurring in old age but capable of striking people in middle age or even younger. The current upsurge in this disease is probably a result of the aging population; fewer people lived long enough to contract this disease in the past. Men are more likely to contract this disease than women in a ratio of 3:2. Variations of the disease and its symptoms are known as Parkinsonism, paralysis agitans, and shaking palsy.

Parkinson's targets a section of the midbrain known as the *substantia nigra*. This section contains neurons that generate dopamine, a neurotransmitter like serotonin, but one that is chiefly responsible for transmitting messages about muscle movement. In patients with Parkinson's disease, the substantia nigra degenerates precipitously, causing the dopamine-generating neurons to die off. As dopamine is necessary for transmitting messages governing motor function, a loss of this neurotransmitter results in tremors, palsy, muscle weaknesses, and a large variety of other physical, mental, and emotional symptoms.

Patients can experience a loss of up to 80% of substantia nigra cells and still function well mentally and physically, so often Parkinson's disease is well advanced before significant outward symptoms manifest themselves. For this reason, the disease usually remains undetected until after 80% of this critical section of the midbrain is already gone.

What are the symptoms of Parkinson's disease?

The early symptoms include mild tremors of the hands (both in action and at rest) and nodding of the head. Movement is progressively slower and harder for the patient to perform. Next, loss of muscle control in the face results in lack of facial expression creating a lifeless, masklike appearance. As the disease advances, the patient may stare vacantly, his mouth dropped open and drooling, blinking uncontrollably, his back bent over—all outward symptoms of "old age" that are really symptoms of a specific, age-related disease.

The disease progresses as more of the substantia nigra dies off and its critical output of the neurotransmitter dopamine slows to a near standstill. The result is seen in a general slowing down of both motor and mental functions. At the motor level, this means a hesitant, shuffling gait as the patient loses his ability to start and stop voluntary movements. Involuntary movements—tremors, ticklike twisting of the wrist and fingers, and shaking of the head—increase substantially. The ability to project one's voice beyond a whisper slips away as does speed of articulation. And the ability to properly hold and guide a pen or pencil slips away too, causing handwriting to go out of control. In general, the whole body stiffens as a result of muscular rigidity, with concomitant muscle pain, especially in the back. Finally, Parkinson's disease patients complain of sleep disturbances and sexual dysfunction.

At the mental level, Parkinson's patients experience significantly slower and less acute thinking functions. But it is the emotional component of this disease that is most devastating. Patients may experience psychosis-like symptoms such as extreme paranoia and hallucinations. But it is serious depression that is the most common and distressing mental consequence of this disease. Parkinson's-related depression manifests itself in general anxiety, severe loss of confidence and self-esteem, and apathy as well as the typical low, pessimistic mood of depression accompanying a loss of will to live. Obviously, much of this depression is a consequence of the other symptoms of the disease: It is truly depressing to suffer such an uncompromising deficit of functions. But there is clearly a depressant component to the disease itself that is related to the decreased output of neurotransmitters. Almost half of all Parkinson's disease patients suffer from severe depression.

What is the cause of Parkinson's disease?

In some cases, the disease is caused by a viral infection of the brain and in some cases of this, the external cause may possibly be environmental toxins, such as carbon monoxide poisoning. Some physicians believe that cerebral arteriosclerosis may contribute to the onset of Parkinson's disease by reducing the blood supply to the substantia nigra, but there is no clear evidence of this.

The bottom line is that although we know a great deal about how this disease behaves in the body, we currently do not know what its general cause is or how to avoid this cause.

EIGHTEEN

The Most Common Treatments for Parkinson's Disease

What are the most commonly prescribed treatments for Parkinson's disease?

Basically, treatment addresses the disease by making up for the substantia nigra's diminished capacity for generating the crucial neurotransmitter dopamine. The primary way it does this is by adding a precursor of dopamine to the system. This precursor, the amino acid dihydroxyphenylalanine (DOPA), manages to get production of dopamine going again, although for a limited period of time. DOPA most frequently is delivered in two forms, levodopa (L-dopa) or carbidopa, the latter enhancing the effects of the former, so physicians often titrate some combination of these two depending on the Parkinson's patient's responses. Some physicians add dopamine "enhancers" such as bromocriptine and pergolide to the mix. In effect, these dopamine enhancers boost the power and speed of the existing population of this neurotransmitter.

Unfortunately, it needs to be stressed that DOPA treatment does not address the underlying degenerative process of Parkinson's disease: It never stops it, nor reverses it. DOPA treatment simply makes up for its most devastating deficit caused by the disease: reduced production of dopamine and all that follows from that.

It also needs to be stressed that DOPA treatment decreases in efficacy over time. Dosage can be increased to try to counter this, but ultimately DOPA treatment stops increasing production of dopamine altogether and the disease takes over from there.

Are there any side effects to DOPA treatment?

Yes, it appears to make Parkinson's patients even more prone to depression. And considering that depression is one of Parkinson's disease's most debilitating mental consequences, this is a very serious side effect indeed. The reason that DOPA increases a patient's vulnerability to depression is probably because this drug depletes our natural SAMe levels, reason enough to complement DOPA treatment with SAMe supplements, as many doctors are now doing.

Other, less frequent side effects include nausea, drop in blood pressure, and hallucinations. Another side effect that has resulted in some embarrassing situations in hospitals and nursing homes is that it appears to act as an aphrodisiac in some men.

Are there any other conventional treatments for Parkinson's disease?

Yes, but in general the other medicinal treatments are less effective than DOPA treatment. On the theory that the cause of the disease is a viral infection of the midbrain, some doctors prescribe the antiviral agent amantadine for Parkinson's patients, but the results of this treatment are inconclusive at best.

Other doctors have prescribed antidepressants—specifically, MAO inhibitors—to address Parkinson's associated depression. As you may recall, the MAO inhibitors boost levels of the neurotransmitter norepinephrine, and thus not only reduce depression but can raise motor activity in Parkinson's patients. This is all good news. But the downside of MAO inhibitors, especially the dangers they present in combination with certain foods and other medications, is familiar to us from Chapter 3.

Finally, surgical options for this disease address Parkinson's at its root, the substantia nigra in the midbrain. The best known and most controversial of these procedures is transplanting fetal substantia nigra brain cells into the brains of Parkinson's disease patients; these still-growing cells then rebuild the damaged substantia nigra in the patient with the end result of resumed function and production of dopamine. The controversy surrounding this procedure has to do with the procurement of the fetal cells themselves—they come from aborted fetuses. But there is another more practical controversy involved here too. Brain surgery is risky in the best of circumstances, but in the case of the great majority of Parkinson's patients it is even more so because they are older people with decreased recuperative abilities.

Another promising surgical approach to Parkinson's disease involves transplanting cloned dopamine-generating animal cells to the patient's brain. No ethical controversy here, but the risks of brain surgery remain the same.

Finally, it should be noted that recent research on brain stem cells—cells that have the potential to regenerate any organs—suggest that regrowth of the substantia nigra may be an option in the not too distant future.

Does alternative medicine offer any promising treatments for Parkinson's disease?

Currently, the drug of choice for many alternative medical practitioners is an over-the-counter (in some health food stores) preparation called deprenyl. Known primarily as a "smart drug" (nootropic) and life extender, deprenyl is similar to MAO inhibitors in its effects, without the codietary dangers of prescription MAO inhibitors.

Advocates of deprenyl treatment for Parkinson's disease claim that the drug not only enhances activity in the substantia nigra, but protects against age-related degeneration of this section of the brain and of the dopaminergic (dopamine-producing) nervous system in general. It is said to inhibit downgrading of several neurotransmitters and to boost the release of dopamine in particular. In this regard, it is similar to DOPA treatment; indeed, proponents of deprenyl treatment say that if Parkinson's patients are treated in an early enough stage of the disease, DOPA treatment may never be necessary. For this reason, some alternative doctors recommend deprenyl as a hedge against Parkinson's disease in older patients. Also, because DOPA treatment is time-limited in effectiveness, these doctors recommend using deprenyl as a way of postponing DOPA treatment until absolutely necessary.

Deprenyl advocates claim that not only does the drug slow down the progression of Parkinson's disease, it improves such symptoms as sluggish thinking and impaired memory and reaction time. At the physical level, it is said to improve motor function and raise the libido. What is more, it is said to be an highly effective antidepressant.

Unfortunately, deprenyl treatment for Parkinson's disease has not been thoroughly enough researched for all of these promising claims to be substantiated. Further, some anecdotal evidence suggests that there may be some seriously unwelcome side effects accompanying this drug, but this too is unsubstantiated. At this point, a wait-and-see attitude is all that can be recommended.

Another alternative medical option, cryosurgery (using a freezing probe) of the brain, is being used in some parts of Europe to reduce the incidence of tremors associated with the disease. Some doctors are experimenting with electrical stimulation of the brain to stimulate the substantia nigra. And still others are experimenting with oxygen treatment in hyperbaric chambers. The jury is still out on all three of these experimental procedures.

Finally, as with osteoarthritis and fibromyalgia, activity is recommended, especially low-impact exercises provided in yoga. At the very least, these can slow the process of the muscle stiffness associated with Parkinson's disease. As well, psychological therapy can help in reducing the stress and depression that invariably accompany this disease.

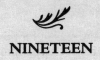

NINETEEN

The SAMe Treatment for Parkinson's Disease

How does SAMe treat Parkinson's disease?

With mixed results. On the one hand, studies have proven that Parkinson's patients have significantly lower levels of SAMe than the normal population. This, of course, leads many scientists to believe that the SAMe deficiency is an unhealthy byproduct of the disease, one that would benefit the patients by being corrected. But, as we will see, this is not necessarily so. In fact, quite the opposite may be true.

On the other hand, other studies have shown that SAMe treatment of Parkinson's patients helps improve both depression and cognitive functions, as well as relieving muscle spasms and tremors.

Let's look at the cautionary evidence first. Several animal studies have demonstrated that injecting the brain with SAMe actually produces symptoms of Parkinson's disease—symptoms like muscle rigidity and tremors. And the reason for this appears to be that a superabundance of SAMe in the brain depletes dopamine—in other words, it has the same effect on this vital neurotransmitter that Parkinson's disease has. Thus, some scientists have theorized that the reason Parkinson's patients have lower levels of SAMe than others is that their bodies are striving to conserve dopamine—that it is a compensatory response of the diseased body rather than part of the disease itself.

But other researchers have come to the conclusion that the lowered levels of SAMe in Parkinson's patients is what causes the severe depression associated with this disease. Obviously, this does not contradict the above theory; lowered levels of SAMe in the brain may both be compensatory when it comes to dopamine production and still add to depression. Perhaps the discrepancy between these two schools of thought comes down to the amount of dosage: While not enough SAMe in the brain has debilitating effects, too much has debilitating effects also.

Fortunately, SAMe treatment for Parkinson's disease has been tested in some thorough studies, both as a treatment on its own and in conjunction with DOPA treatments. And the results are very encouraging. One recent double-blind study reported in *Current Therapeutic Research* demonstrated relief from depression in only two weeks for 72 % of Parkinson's patients treated with SAMe. Another study at Beth Israel Hospital in New York confirmed these results, with many of the test subjects going from severe chronic depression to no depression at all. (Incidently, patients in this study were given doses of SAMe up to 3,300 mg per day.) In some ongoing studies, the additional benefits of reduced tremors and muscle spasms are being reported.

Finally, studies of Parkinson's patients who are currently being treated with DOPA show some very promising results. First, SAMe treatment in no way interferes with the effects of the DOPA; in fact, some evidence suggests that SAMe supplements actually improves the response of Parkinson's patients to DOPA treatment. This, in turn, has led some doctors to believe that if SAMe is added, they can prescribe lower doses of DOPA with the end result that DOPA treatment can work for a longer period of time. And second, as DOPA has the unwelcome side effect of causing or deepening depression in Parkinson's patients, the addition of SAMe to the regime will counteract this unfortunate effect.

In short, SAMe is at this point only a very promising treatment for Parkinson's disease on its own. It does not go to the cause of the disease and it addresses only some of its symptoms. But from all the evidence, SAMe is a worthwhile supplement to treatment with DOPA and should be considered by all Parkinson's patients who are currently using or are planning to use DOPA treatment.

PART VI

SAMe and Alzheimer's Disease

TWENTY

What Is Alzheimer's Disease and Who Gets It?

What is Alzheimer's disease?

Alzheimer's disease is a progressive form of dementia (deterioration of mental functions) that strikes 6% of people over the age of 65, with that percentage growing rapidly in older age groups. As our population survives other fatal ailments (heart disease and cancer) in greater numbers, this devastating disease strikes an increasingly higher percentage of our aging population, causing the National Institute of Aging to deem it the number one problem of older people. It strikes slightly more women than men (although this statistic may represent the simple fact that women live longer than men) and appears to have a genetic component, with direct relations of Alzheimer's patients more likely to contract the disease in a ratio of 4:1.

What are the symptoms of Alzheimer's disease?

First and foremost, Alzheimer's patients lose their memories, in particular their short-term memories. But as the disease progresses, all memory slips away, including the ability to recognize and remember one's closest relatives and loved ones. As part of this loss, word recall, including the ability to remember the names of people and objects, drops away too (this is called anomic aphasia). This thorough loss of memory has cataclysmic effects on the personality and identity of the patient. In a sense, the sum of our personal memories is who we are, so without these memories, our very selves slip away.

Many of the personality changes in Alzheimer's patients are reflected in their behavior, which is often inappropriate. This includes foul language and juvenile and crude humor, appearing naked in public, sudden and violent outbursts, and slovenliness.

Alzheimer's patients also experience severe spatial difficulties ranging from general disorientation to the inability to gauge the size and shape of objects tactilely. As in osteoarthritis, fibromyalgia, and Parkinson's disease, advanced Alzheimer's patients develop rigidity in their legs and arms and have difficulty walking. In the final stages of this disease, seizures—some of them fatal—occur. The average course of the disease from onset to death is five years, the general range being one to ten years.

Currently, there are no tests for definitively diagnosing Alzheimer's disease. However, the course of the disease can be monitored indirectly by imaging the progressive atrophy of the brain with MRIs and/or CAT scans. These tests could be revealing other, unrelated and possibly treatable types of dementia, so diagnosis of Alzheimer's disease is often a process of exclusion or elimination—that is, if symptoms do not respond to treatments for these other types of dementia, a diagnosis of Alzheimer's disease is made.

What is the cause of Alzheimer's disease?

At this time, the primary cause of Alzheimer's is unknown. What we do know is that the disease directly results in significantly reduced amounts of neurotransmitters in the brain. Further, all attempts to artificially boost the dwindling population of neurotransmitters neither reduces the progression of the disease nor seems to significantly reverse its symptoms.

Currently, however, there are a number of theories as to the cause of this disease, some of them strikingly similar to the theories as to the cause of Parkinson's disease. One such theory is that free radical cell damage is the root of this disease; thus the reason that it strikes older people is that the accumulation of free radicals and their cumulative destruction increases as the immune systems age and break down. Another theory is that the disease is a byproduct of arteriosclerosis; blood flow to the brain is reduced resulting in accelerated brain cell death. Still another theory puts the blame on the hormone imbalances that come with age. Among these, a Stanford Medical School researcher suggests that stress and the stress-induced hormone cortisol are fundamental causes of the brain deterioration associated with Alzheimer's.

Another scientist suggests that inadequate calcium regulation within the brain cells is the root cause. And some theorists believe that Alzheimer's is yet another result of environmental toxins including iron and lead, but especially singling out aluminum. Finally, there is the cholinergic theory, which posits a breakdown of the cholinergic neurotransmitter system as the basic cause, cholinergics being nerve fibers that liberate acetylcholine at brain-neuron connection points.

So what we are left with are several theories, most of which do not necessarily contradict the other (the disease may have several causes) and none of which is currently provable.

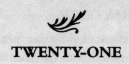

TWENTY-ONE

Treatments for Alzheimer's Disease

What are the most commonly prescribed treatments for Alzheimer's disease?

Although currently there are a variety of treatments in various stages of experimental development, at this date there is no consensus in the traditional medical community on how to treat Alzheimer's disease. Certainly, without a known cause, it is virtually impossible to find a cure. And, as noted in Chapter 20, various attempts to relieve symptoms of this disease by artificially boosting the dwindling population of neurotransmitters neither reduces the progression of the disease nor seems to significantly reverse its symptoms.

Recently, the FDA approved a drug called tacrine (brand name Cognex) for use with Alzheimer's patients. It addresses some of the cognitive deficit with modest results. It also packs a wallop in unwelcome side effects, including diarrhea, vomiting, loss of appetite, fainting, and skin rashes. But with no substantial alternatives around, it is currently the drug of choice by many traditional doctors.

When it comes to prevention of the disease, some studies show hope for various preventative treatments. High on this list are daily small doses of the anti-inflammatory ibuprofen. How this mitigates against onset of Alzheimer's disease is not specifically known, but controlled studies convincingly demonstrate that ibuprofen-taking groups show a markedly lower incidence of Alzheimer's than control groups. As we have noted, one study suggests that the stress hormone cortisol is at the root of the cognitive problems associated with the disease, so long-range prevention should include a low-stress lifestyle. (This, of course, is a prescription for reducing the possibility of most diseases, particularly those related to the immune system.) Finally, following from the toxin theory of Alzheimer's cause, prevention includes avoiding excessive intake of lead, iron, and particularly aluminum, which has definitely been associated with brain cell damage. To go along with the non–aluminum prevention regime, one must eschew aluminum and aluminum-containing cookware and beauty products, and aluminum-buffered aspirin and antacids, among other products.

Does alternative medicine offer any Alzheimer's treatments?

Yes, a great many. But again, the majority of alternative treatments for Alzheimer's disease remain untested.

Most alternative treatments center around supplements of various kinds, ranging from common vitamins (the B vitamins, including folic acid, and vitamins C and E) and minerals (particularly zinc and magnesium) to several over-the-counter "smart drugs" (nootropics). Let's take a look at three of the most often recommended and most promising nootropics.

Ginkgo biloba. A natural extract of the tree by the same name, ginkgo biloba is an ancient folk medicine that recently has been convincingly proven to increase blood flow to the extremities and now is frequently prescribed for peripheral vascular diseases. Ginkgo also has been proven to increase blood flow to the brain and therefore is used to improve brain function. In one double-blind study of patients over age 50 who suffered from mild to moderate memory impairment, a three-times-a-day dosage of ginkgo biloba measurably improved not only short-term memory, but other cognitive functions, including speed of learning new material and reaction times. But more significantly, a controlled study that was published in the prestigious *Journal of the American Medical Association* demonstrated that 40 mg of ginkgo biloba administered orally three times a day (with meals) significantly improved cognitive functions in Alzheimer's patients. A bonus: Ginkgo also appears to improve mood in mild and moderate depressives. Normal dosages of this relatively inexpensive supplement range from 150 mg per day (in three 50 mg doses) to 600 mg per day (in three 200 mg doses).

Acetyl-L-Carnitine. Acetyl-L-Carnitine is a synthetic, acetylated version of the naturally occurring L-Carnitine, a substance that enhances ATP (energy-storing molecules) production in the mitochondria. A variety of animal and human studies have amply demonstrated that this synthetic L-Carnitine prevents age-related lipid peroxidation of brain cells and reduction in nerve growth factor. They also show that Acetyl-L-Carnitine protects receptors in the hippocampus area of the brain from free radicals.

A great number of well-designed studies with both normal subjects and those suffering from Alzheimer's disease have shown that both groups experienced improvement in memory, attention levels, and reflex speed while taking moderate doses of Acetyl-L-Carnitine. But the most impressive results for Alzheimer's patients came from a 1992 study that found that in addition to improved cognitive functions people with this disease who received 2,000 mg of Acetyl-L-Carnitine per day over the course of a year experienced a significant reduction in the progress of the disease compared with a control group. This fact alone is sufficient for some patients to add Acetyl-L-Carnitine to their regime as a hedge against further deterioration. General dosage ranges from 500 to 2,000 mg per day, with the higher amount recommended to start with. Note: Acetyl-L-Carnitine is currently very expensive.

Deprenyl. As you may recall from the section on Parkinson's disease, deprenyl protects against age-related degeneration of various sections of the brain and of the dopaminergic (dopamine-producing) nervous system in general. It is said to inhibit downgrading of several neurotransmitters and to boost the release of dopamine in particular.

A statistically significant number of double-blind studies have demonstrated that 5 to 10 mg of deprenyl twice a day improves memory, attention, language (verbal memory) abilities, sustained concentration, and visuospatial abilities in Alzheimer's patients. The authors of one of these studies noted that the drug "improved information processing abilities and learning strategies at the moment of acquisition" in Alzheimer's patients. And one other doctor stated unequivocally, "Alzheimer's disease patients need to be treated daily with 10 mg of deprenyl from diagnosis until death. Period."

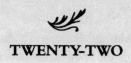

TWENTY-TWO

SAMe Treatment for Alzheimer's Disease

How does SAMe treat Alzheimer's disease?

Unfortunately, it is hard to say because the test results are scant at this time. This is why I have saved Alzheimer's treatment for the last chapter in this book: The evidence that SAMe helps is promising, but inconclusive. But let's look at the promising evidence.

First, it has been amply demonstrated that SAMe concentrations in the entire body decrease with age and this decrease appears to be totally unrelated to diet deficiencies. Further, autopsies of patients with Alzheimer's disease demonstrate conclusively that, compared to the non-Alzheimer's population, Alzheimer's patients show a significantly lower concentration of SAMe in their brains. We only have theories of why this is so. Either it is because there is diminished production of SAMe in Alzheimer's patient's brains, increased (compensatory) use of SAMe by the brain, or both. As we saw in our discussion of SAMe and Parkinson's disease, these low levels of SAMe in the brain do not necessarily mean that this deficiency is part of the disease, but it does make this a promising hypothesis that suggests adding SAMe to the patient's diet is beneficial.

Next, we have indirect evidence that SAMe can benefit Alzheimer's patients because it increases permeability of cell membranes. As you may recall, this effect of SAMe is crucial in its treatment of depression, osteoarthritis, and cirrhosis of the liver, so there is good reason to believe that it would have the same effect on the permeability of brain cell membranes. What can be proven is that SAMe supplements definitely increase the density of critical brain receptors with the result of increased brain activity and cognitive function. But again, unfortunately, there have not been a sufficient number of controlled studies showing if this effect is operative in Alzheimer's patients.

This does not seem like an awful lot to go on as far as treatment with SAMe for Alzheimer's patients. Yet given the paucity of alternatives, many respectable doctors add modest SAMe dosage to the medical regime of Alzheimer's patients as a calculated bet.

Can SAMe be taken with other Alzheimer's disease medications?

Yes. Again, the only risk is economic. But in the face of no reasonable alternatives, many doctors prescribe a regime of Acetyl-L-Carnitine, deprenyl, and SAMe, taken concurrently.

Ongoing and future research into this dreaded disease will in time turn up better and more dependable treatments. SAMe may very well be an integral part of these future treatments.

Appendix A
Buying SAMe

As with all unregulated over-the-counter supplements and drugs, quality of the product varies. In fact, one cannot always be sure from the information on the label how much of the active ingredients of SAMe are actually in a particular product. Until recently, all SAMe came in the relatively unstable toslyate form, but now a much more stable form called butanedsulfonate is available from Nature Made and GNC, and these are the products most frequently recommended by doctors. Finally, SAMe, like aspirin, is basically absorbed in the intestine, so to ensure it reaches the intestine intact it is best taken in (enteric) coated tablets.

As we've noted earlier, SAMe is relatively expensive, but even these relatively high prices do vary, from $2.50 per 400 mg dose to $18.50 for the same dose.

Here is a rundown of current prices per 400 mg dose of the most available and dependable brands of coated SAMe tablets*

Nature Made	$2.50 ($1.90 on the Internet)
GNC	$3.00
NutraLife	$3.20 ($2.20 in bulk)
Life Extension	$4.50 ($3.34 in bulk)
Solgar	$5.40

---

*For updated price and quality information, consult the SAMe consumer pricing guide on the Worldwide Web: *http://www.immunesupport.com/compare.htm*

Appendix B
Further Information

BOOKS

For more information about SAMe and depression, the best book for the lay reader is Dr. Richard Brown's *Stop Depression Now* (1999, Putnam). Brown, a professor of psychiatry at Columbia University as well as a psychopharmacologist, has direct clinical experience prescribing SAMe as an antidepressant.

For more information about SAMe and osteoarthritis, the best book for the lay reader is Dr. Sol Grazi's *SAMe* (1999, Prima), a low-key but thorough and thoroughly accessible short book.

WEB SITES

For updated information about SAMe and depression, see: *http://www.psycom.net/depression.central.same.html*

For updated information about SAMe and arthritis, see: *http://www.members.tripod.come/SAMestuff/arthritis.html*

For updated information about SAMe and fibromyalgia, see: *http://www.americanwholehealth.com/library/fibromyalgian/fms32.htm*

Index

A
Accountable bad mood, 15, 16
Acetaminophen
    fibromyalgia and, 152
    osteoarthritis and, 109, 111
Acetylcholine, 214
Acetyl-L-Carnitine (ALC), 52,
    59–60
    Alzheimer's disease and,
        218–19, 223
    side effects, 60
Acupressure
    arthritis, as treatment for,
        118
    fibromyalgia, as treatment for,
        154
Acupuncture
    arthritis, as treatment for, 118,
        130
    fibromyalgia, as treatment for,
        154
ADD see Attention Deficit
    Disorder (ADD)
Adenosine triphosphate (ATP),
    61, 124

Adrenaline, SAMe regulation of,
    64, 161
Advil, 112
Alcohol, 23
    cirrhosis, effect on, 172,
        173–76
    liver, effect on, 171
    SAMe, use of while taking, 86
Alcoholic hepatitis, 176
Aleve, 152
Alexander method
    depression, as treatment for, 42
    fibromyalgia, as treatment for,
        154
    osteoarthritis, as treatment for,
        121
Aluminum, 214, 216
Alzheimer's disease, 2, 68,
    211–14
    Acetyl-L-Carnitine and, 59
    Acetyl-L-Carnitine and
        deprenyl, SAMe taken in
        conjunction with, 223
    alternative treatments, 217
    aluminum and, 214, 216

Alzheimer's disease (*continued*)
CAT scans, 212
cause of, 213–14
cholingeric theory, 214
common treatments for, 215–19
defined, 211
deprenyl and Acetyl-L-Carnitine, SAMe taken in conjunction with, 223
deprenyl as treatment for, 219, 223
MRI, 212
nootropics and, 217
SAMe, 65, 221–23
Acetyl-L-Carnitine and deprenyl, taken in conjunction with, 223
symptoms of, 212
toxin theory, 214, 216
vitamin C and, 217
vitamin E and, 217
Amantadine, 201
Amebic dysentery, 176
American Psychiatric Association
bad mood, reasonable cause for, 19
definition of depression, 16
statistics on depression, 25
Amitriptyline, 46
Ammonia poisoning, 180, 181
Anafranil (clomipramine), 157
Analgesics
fibromyalgia and, 151
osteoarthritis, as treatment for, 109, 110–11
Anomic aphasia, 212
Antidepressants, 45–49
natural, 51–60
prescription, 45–49
Anxiety disorders
5-HTP and, 64
kava-kava and, 56, 64
L-tryptophan and, 64

melatonin and, 64
SAMe and, 64
valerian root and, 57, 64
yoga and, 35
Arteriosclerosis, 213
Arthritis, 95–107
CAT scans, 107
defined, 95
gout, 100
osteoarthritis *see* Osteoarthritis
rheumatoid arthritis, 96–99, 106
septic arthritis, 99–100
tests to determine, 106–7
Arthroscopy, 116, 129
Aspirin
chondrocytes, effect on, 129
fibromyalgia and, 151, 152
osteoarthritis, as treatment for, 109, 110–11
side effects, 112
ATP *see* Adenosine triphosphate (ATP)
Attention Deficit Disorder (ADD), 148

B
Bad mood
American Psychiatric Association's reasonable cause for, 19
depression distinguished from, 15–17
reasonable cause for, 19
Beck Depression Inventory, 162
Beta carotene, free radicals and, 125
Bile, 170, 175
Bioenergetics, 42
Bipolar disorder, 27, 68
SAMe and, 27, 70
Body weight, excessive, 104–5
Body work therapies, 42
Bromocriptine, 199

C
Calcium, osteoarthritis and, 122
Carbidopa, 199
Cartilage, 95–96
  breakdown of, 104
CAT scans
  Alzheimer's disease, in, 212
  arthritis and, 107
  fibromyalgia and, 146
  osteoarthritis and, 133
Celexa (citalopram), 48
Cerebral arteriosclerosis, 198
Chondrocytes, 103, 114, 125, 126, 128, 129
Chronic depression, 14
  SAMe and, 70
  treatments for, 33
  yoga and, 35
Chronic fatigue syndrome, 144, 147
Cirrhosis, 2, 171–76
  alcohol, effect of, 172, 173–76
  ammonia poisoning, 180, 181
  common treatments for, 179–81
  conventional treatments, SAMe compared with, 186
  hepatitis as symptom of, 176
  SAMe, 183–91
    conventional treatments, compared with, 186
    dosage suggestions, 190
    efficacy, evidence of, 187–88
    other therapies, in conjunction with, 186–87
    relief, time before feeling, 191
  symptoms of, 172–73
  vitamin B_{12} and, 187–90
  vitamin E and, 172
Cloprednol, 98
Cocaine, 23
Cognex, 215
Colchicine, 100
Collagen, 103, 126, 128

Cortisone, 116, 129
Cryosurgery, 203–4
Cushing's syndrome, 116, 129

D
Deprenyl, 60
  Alzheimer's disease and, 219, 223
  Parkinson's disease, 202–3
Depression, 2, 6, 7
  acknowledgment of, 30
  American Psychiatric Association definition of, 16
  American Psychiatric Association statistics on, 25
  antidepressants, 45–49
  bad mood distinguished, 15–17
  behavioral symptoms, 14
  cause of, 20
  chemistry of, 21
  contagious aspect of, 26
  defined, 13
  degrees of, 14–15
  demographic statistics, 29
  diet and lifestyle, effect of, 36
  effect on other people, 25–26
  exercise as treatment for, 35
  fibromyalgia, as symptom of, 144, 156–57
  Freudian psychologists' view of, 20
  genetic predisposition to, 21–22
  Parkinson's-related depression, 197
  pharmacological therapies for, 43–60
  physical cause of, 20
  psychological therapies for, 39–42
  SAMe
    dosage suggestions, 78–81
    duration of treatment, 84

Depression (*continued*)
    effectiveness of, 69–70
    fast-action approach, 79–81
    meta-analyses of studies, 72–75
    other antidepressants, used in conjunction with, 76–78
    relationship between, 62
    relief, time before feeling, 66–67
    SSRIs and, 77
    St. John's wort combined with, 78
    studies detailing, 66–67, 72–75
    testing of, 71–75
    as treatment for, 61–92
    tricyclics combined with, 76
  self-medication of, 23
  signs of, 30–31
  SSRIs, SAMe combined with, 77
  St. John's wort, SAMe combined with, 78
  symptoms of, 13–14, 82
  treatments for, 33–37
  tricyclics, SAMe combined with, 76
  types of, 27–29
  vitamin C as treatment for, 36
Desipramine, 46, 70
Diet and lifestyle
  depression, treatment for, 36
  osteoarthritis, treatment for, 118–22, 130–31
Dihydroxyphenylalanine (DOPA) treatment, 199
  SAMe, in conjunction with, 206–7
  side effects, 200
DNA methylation, 5, 63, 184
Dopamine, 44, 62, 63, 161, 199, 206
  MAO inhibitors and, 47

  St. John's wort and, 52
  substantia nigra and, 195
Dopamine enhancers, 199
Dopaminergic nervous system, 202, 219
DOPA treatment *see* Dihydroxyphenylalanine (DOPA) treatment
Doxepin, 46

E
ECT *see* Electroconvulsive therapy (ECT)
Effexor (venlafaxine), 48
Elavil (amitriptyline), 157
Electroconvulsive therapy (ECT)
  as treatment for chronic depression, 33
Electromyography (EMG), 146
EMG *see* Electromyography (EMG)
Erythrocytes, 169
Erythrocyte sedimentation rate test (ESR), 106, 107
ESR *see* Erythrocyte sedimentation rate test (ESR)
Estrogen, osteoarthritis and, 104, 127
Exercise
  depression, as treatment for, 35
  fibromyalgia and, 154
  osteoarthritis, as benefit to, 131

F
Fatigue, 35, 43, 87
  depression, as symptom of, 14
Fibromyalgia, 2, 68, 143–49
  acupressure as treatment for, 154
  Alexander method, 154
  CAT scans, 146
  causes of, 149
  common treatments for, 151–58
  defined, 143
  depression, role of, 156–57

diagnosing, 146–47
exercise and, 154
Halcion, 153
MRI, 144
psychological therapy as
    treatment for, 158
SAMe, 159–65
    depression, countering,
        160–62
    dosage suggestions, 164
    studies of, 162–63
shiatsu as treatment for, 154
sleeping aids for, 152–53
stress reduction, importance of,
    154–56
symptoms of, 144–46
Tender Point Examination, 147
Transcendental Meditation and,
    155
x rays, 144, 146
yoga as treatment for, 154, 155
5-HTP, 52, 57–59
anxiety disorders and, 64
fibromyalgia and, 153
side effects, 58
Flexeril, 152
Folic acid
    Alzheimer's disease and, 217
    cirrhosis and, 179, 187
    osteoarthritis and, 122, 131
    SAMe production, 66
Free radicals, 127
    Alzheimer's disease, 213
    cirrhosis and, 184, 188
    defined, 125
Freudian psychologists' view of
    depression, 20
Frontal lobotomy, 33

G
Gallstones, 172
Gastritis, 112
Ginkgo biloba, 60
    Alzheimer's disease and,
        217–18

Glutathione, 5, 124–25, 127, 160,
    184, 189
Glycogen, 170
Gonococcus, 99
Gout, 100
Green algae, 1
Gristle, 95
Gulf War syndrome, 147

H
Halcion, 153
HAM-d *see* Hamilton Depression
    Scale (HAM-D)
Hamilton Depression Scale
    (HAM-D), 72, 82
Hand gyms, 120
Healing magnets, 118
Hemophilus influenza, 99
Hepatitis, 172
    common treatments for,
        181–82
    defined, 176
    SAMe as treatment for, 191
    vitamin C as treatment for, 182
Homocysteine, 5
Hypertension, MAO inhibitors
    and, 47

I
Ibuprofen, 109, 112
    Alzheimer's disease, 216
    SAMe compared to, 136
Imipramine, 46
Infectious hepatitis, 176
Injuries, osteoarthritis and, 106
Insomnia, 35, 43, 49, 87
    depression, as symptom of, 14
    kava-kava and, 56
Interferon, 181
Isocarboxazid, 47

J
Jaundice, 173
Joint replacement surgery, 116,
    129

K
Kava-kava (*Piper methysticum*), 52, 55–56
    anxiety disorders and, 56, 64
    fibromyalgia and, 153, 156
    side effects, 56
Kidneys, NSAIDs' effect on, 113

L
L-dopa *see* Levodopa (L-dopa)
Levodopa (L-dopa), 199
L-glutathione, free radicals and, 125
Lifestyle *see* Diet and lifestyle
Limbic cycle, 149
Liver, 169–77
    alcohol and, 171
    defined, 169
    detoxifier, as, 170
    diseases of *see* Cirrhosis; Hepatitis
    NSAIDs damaging, 113, 114
    regenerating quality of, 170
    SAMe, relationship with, 183–85
    transplants, 181
L-tryptophan, 52, 57–59
    anxiety disorders and, 64
    side effects, 58
Luvox (fluvoxamine), 48

M
Magnesium
    cirrhosis and, 179, 187
    osteoarthritis and, 122, 131
Magnetic resonance imaging (MRI), 106–7, 137
    Alzheimer's disease, in, 212
    fibromyalgia and, 144
Manic-depressive syndrome, 27
MAO inhibitors *see* Monoamine oxidase (MAO) inhibitors
Massage therapy, 42, 117, 130
Master antioxidant *see* Glutathione
Medical journals, bias of, 7

Meditation, 35
Melatonin, 1, 52, 53–55, 62, 161
    anxiety disorders and, 64
    fibromyalgia and, 153
    side effects, 55
Methionine, 65, 124, 184
Methylation, 61, 63, 124, 161
    defined, 3, 5
Minoxidil, 4
Mitochondria, 174, 189
Moderate depression, 15
    SAMe and, 70
    yoga and, 35
Monoamine oxidase (MAO) inhibitors, 47–48
    Parkinson's disease, treatment for, 201
    SAMe, interaction with, 86, 140, 164
Mononucleosis, 176
Mood diary, 82, 91–92
Motrin, 112
MRI *see* Magnetic resonance imaging (MRI)

N
Naproxen, 109, 112
    SAMe compared to, 135
National Institute of Aging, 211
Natural antidepressants, 51–60
Neurotransmitters
    defined, 44
    SAMe's effect on, 62–64
Nonsteroidal anti-inflammatories (NSAIDs), 109, 111–15, 127
    blood thinning side effects, 113
    fibromyalgia and, 151, 152
    gastrointestinal side effects, 112–13
Nonverbal psychological therapy, 41–42
Nootropics, 59, 60
    Alzheimer's disease and, 217
    Parkinson's disease, 202

Norepinephrine, 44
  MAO inhibitors and, 47, 201
  St. John's wort and, 52
  tricyclics and, 46
Norpamin (desipramine), 157
Nortriptyline, 46
NSAIDs *see* Nonsteroidal anti-
    inflammatories (NSAIDs)

O
Orgone Box, Wilhelm Reich's, 42
Osteoarthritis, 2, 6, 7, 67, 95, 130
  acupressure, 118
  acupuncture, 118, 130
  alternative therapies, 117–18
  alternative treatments, SAMe
      compared with, 130
  analgesics, SAMe compared
      with, 128–29
  calcium and, 122, 131
  CAT scans, 133
  causes of, 102–6
  chemistry of, 126–27
  climate, effect of, 121–22
  common treatments for,
      109–22
  conventional treatments, SAMe
      compared with, 128–29
  diet and lifestyle, effect of,
      118–22, 130–31
  exercise as benefit to, 131
  folic acid and, 122, 131
  free radicals, 125
  hand gyms, 120
  healing magnets, 118
  heat therapy, 117, 130
  magnesium and, 122, 131
  massage therapy, 117, 130
  medical tests for, 106–7
  NSAIDs, SAMe compared
      with, 128–29
  potassium and, 122, 131
  SAMe, 123–40
    alternative treatments,
        compared with, 130

  conventional treatments,
      compared with, 128–29
    as cure, 123
    dosage suggestions, 138–39
    relief, time before feeling,
        140
    studies of, 132–37
  shiatsu, 118
  steroids, SAMe compared with,
      129
  surgery, SAMe compared with,
      129
  surgical procedures, 110,
      116–17
  Swedish massage, 118
  symptoms of, 101–2
  tai chi and, 120
  transcutaneous electrical nerve
      stimulation (TENS), 118
  vitamin B_{12} and, 120, 131
  vitamin C and, 122, 131
  yoga and, 120, 131
Over-the-counter remedies, 51–52

P
Pancreatitis, 172
Paralysis agitans, 195
Parkinsonism, 195
Parkinson's disease, 2, 68, 195–98
  alternative treatments, 202–4
  cause of, 198
  common treatments for,
      199–204
  defined, 195
  demographics of, 195
  DOPA treatment, in
      conjunction with SAMe,
      206–7
  nootropics and, 202
  SAMe, 65
    DOPA treatment, in
        conjunction with, 206–7
    studies of, 205–7
  symptoms of, 196–98
  yoga as treatment for, 204

Paxil (paroxetine), 48
Pergolide, 199
Pharmaceutical companies, bias of, 8
Pharmacological therapies for depression, 43–60
  natural types of, 51–60
  prescription types of, 45–49
Phenelzine, 47
Phosphates, 179, 187
Phospholipid methylation, 63, 161, 184
Potassium, osteoarthritis and, 122, 131
Prednisone, 109, 116, 129
Premenstrual syndrome (PMS), 27
  SAMe and, 28–29
Prescription antidepressants, 45–49
Primal scream therapy, 42
Prostaglandins, 110, 112, 113
Protein methylation, 63, 184
Proteoglycan, 103, 114, 125, 126, 128, 129
Prothrombin, 170
Prozac (fluoxetine), 48, 85
  cost of, 85
  SAMe compared to, 4
  side effects of, 4
Psychological therapy *see also* Talk therapy
  fibromyalgia, as treatment for, 158
  nonverbal, 41–42
  SAMe used in conjunction with, 87–91
Pyridoxine, 179, 187

R
RAF *see* Rheumatoid arthritis factor blood test (RAF)
Reference materials, additional books, 227
  websites, 228

Religion as treatment for depression, 34
Remethylation, 5
Repetitive motions, osteoarthritis and, 105
Rheumatoid arthritis, 96–99
  tests to determine, 106
Rheumatoid arthritis factor blood test (RAF), 106, 107
Ritalin, 148
Robaxin, 152
Rolfing, 42

S
S-adenosylmethionine *see* SAMe
S-adenosylmethionine synthetase, 184
SAMe
  alternative ways to boost amount of, 65–66
  beneficial effects of, 2–3
  boost amount of, alternative ways to, 65–66
  brand names, 226
  chemistry of, 124–26
  cirrhosis, as treatment for *see* Cirrhosis
  cost of, 85
  depression, as treatment for *see* Depression
  dosage suggestions *see* specific illness
  drug interactions with, 86, 140, 164
  fast-action approach, 79–81
  fibromyalgia, as treatment for *see* Fibromyalgia
  foods high in, 65
  hepatitis, as treatment for, 191
  liver, relationship with, 183–85
  MAO inhibitors, interactions with *see* Monoamine oxidase (MAO) inhibitors

marketing of, 2
methyl donor, as, 5
osteoarthritis, as treatment for
    see Osteoarthritis
overdosing on, 86, 140
Parkinson's disease, as
    treatment for *see*
    Parkinson's disease
prices of, 225–26
psychotherapy, used in
    conjunction with, 87–91
purchasing of, 225–26
scientific testing of, 7–9
Selective serotonin reuptake
    inhibitors (SSRIs),
    combined with, 77
side effects, 67–69
transsulfuration, 124
Seasonal affect disorder, 27
melatonin and, 54
SAMe and, 28
Selective serotonin reuptake
    inhibitors (SSRIs),
    48–49
SAMe combined with, 77
Septic arthritis, 99–100
Serotonin, 44, 62, 63, 161, 195
MAO inhibitors and, 47
St. John's wort and, 52
tricyclics and, 46
Serum hepatitis, 176
vaccine for, 182
Severe depression *see* Chronic
    depression
Shaking palsy, 195
Shark's fin cartilage, 1
Shiatsu, 118
fibromyalgia, as treatment for,
    154
Shock therapy as treatment for
    chronic depression, 33
Single depressive episode, 14
Soporifics, 152
Spiritual counseling as treatment
    for depression, 34

SSRIs *see* Selective serotonin
    reuptake inhibitors
    (SSRIs)
St. John's wort (*Hypericum
    perforatum*), 1, 52–53
cost of, 85
fibromyalgia and, 156
SAMe combined with, 78
side effects, 53
Staphylococcus, 99
Steroids, 115–16
fibromyalgia and, 151, 152
SAMe compared with, 129
Substantia nigra, 195, 196, 199
electrical stimulation of, 204
surgery on, 201–2
Sulindac (Clinoril), 109, 112
Swedish massage, 118

T
Tacrine, 215
Tagamet, 113
Tai chi as treatment for
    osteoarthritis, 120, 131
Talk therapy, 33, 39–41
duration of, 41
Tender Point Examination, 147
TENS *see* Transcutaneous
    electrical nerve
    stimulation (TENS)
Testosterone, osteoarthritis and,
    104, 127
Thiamine, 179, 187
Transcendental Meditation,
    155
Transcutaneous electrical nerve
    stimulation (TENS),
    118
Transference, 40
Transsulfuration, 124
Tranylcypromine, 47
Trauma, osteoarthritis and, 106
Tricyclics, 45–47, 62
SAMe combined with, 76
Tylenol, 111

U
Ulcers, 112
Ultram, 152
Unaccountable bad mood *see*
    Depression

V
Valerian root (*Valeriana
    officinalis*), 52, 57
    anxiety disorders and, 57, 64
    fibromyalgia and, 153
Valium, 57
Vitamin A, cirrhosis and, 172,
    180
Vitamin B$_{12}$
    cirrhosis and, 187–90
    osteoarthritis and, 120, 131
    SAMe production, 66
Vitamin C
    Alzheimer's disease and, 217
    depression, as treatment for, 36
    free radicals and, 125
    hepatitis, as treatment for, 182
    osteoarthritis and, 122, 131
Vitamin D, cirrhosis and, 172
Vitamin E
    Alzheimer's disease and, 217
    cirrhosis and, 172
    free radicals and, 125
Vitamin K, 179, 180, 187

W
Web sites, 228
Weight loss or gain
    depression, as symptom of, 13
    osteoarthritis, as benefit to,
        118–19, 130–31
Wilhelm Reich's Orgone Box, 42

X
X rays, 107, 133
    fibromyalgia and, 144, 146

Y
Yoga
    anxiety disorders and, 35
    depression, as treatment for,
        35
    fibromyalgia, as treatment for,
        154, 155
    osteoarthritis, as treatment for,
        120, 131
    Parkinson's disease, as
        treatment for, 204

Z
Zantac, 113
Zinc, 217
Zoloft (sertraline), 48